THE SUCCESSFUL PRACTICE
IN GOOD TIMES AND BAD

Morton M. Ehudin, DDS

PennWell Books / DENTAL ECONOMICS

Copyright © 1990 by
PennWell Publishing Company
1421 South Sheridan/P.O. Box 1260
Tulsa, Oklahoma 74101

Library of Congress cataloging in publication data/Morton M. Ehudin

Ehudin, Morton M.
The successful dental practice in good times and bad
p. cm.
Includes indes.
ISBN 0-87814-361-0
1. Dentristry — Practice. 2. Dental economics. I. Title.
[DNLM: 1. Practice Management, Dental. WU 77 E336s]
RK58.E395 1990
617.6'0068 — dc20
DNM/DLC
for Library of Congress
90-14235
CIP

Printed in the United States of America

1 2 3 4 5 94 93 92 91 90

Dedicated to:
Albert "Shorty" Ehudin
Who taught me the first Law of Business

With Special Thanks to My Partners:
Colleen, Dottie, Gail, Karen, Lovie, Sherry,
and especially Lynne.

TABLE OF CONTENTS

INTRODUCTION vii

CHAPTER ONE
The Successful Practice of the Future 1

CHAPTER TWO
Riding the Roller Coaster 9

CHAPTER THREE
Putting Your Practice
on a Firm Financial Foundation 17

CHAPTER FOUR
Volume vs. Quality 41

CHAPTER FIVE
Internal / External Marketing 45

CHAPTER SIX
The Dental Team 64

CHAPTER SEVEN
The Hygiene Program –
the Heartbeat of Your Practice 82

CHAPTER EIGHT
Specialties – No Longer so Special 92

CHAPTER NINE
Advanced Planning 98

CHAPTER TEN
Summing Up 102

INTRODUCTION

If you're like me, before you take advice from anyone, you like to know to whom you're listening, what his background is, and what he's up to. If that's not important to you, you can skip this first section and just take what I have to say on pure faith.

Well, I see you're still with me, so here goes:

I did my undergraduate work at the University of Maryland at College Park and came back to Baltimore, where I graduated from the dental school in 1960. Then it was four years in the U.S. Army Dental Corps. I spent three of those four years in Mannheim, Germany, and for two of the three I was the chief of a small clinic in downtown Mannheim. I know that most of my fellow officers thought I was crazy. While they spent most of their time trying to see how little dentistry they could do, I spent mine doing as much as I could. I wasn't sure what they had in mind for the future, but I knew I was going out into private practice, and I wanted to sharpen my skills and get to be fast. So when the guys who worked under me were in the lounge drinking coffee and working the crossword puzzles, I was working two operatories with two assistants and figuring out how to be really efficient.

By the time I sailed home from Europe at the end of 1964, I was chomping at the bit–ready to take on the world. I knew that I wanted to be somewhere in the suburbs of Washington, so I rented an apartment in the area and started looking around for the right spot to open an office. In the meantime, the bills needed to be paid, so I took a position as an associate in a big, busy general practice in southern Maryland. That experience was a real eye-opener! I thought I knew something about dentistry, and I guess I did have some basic skills developed by then; but I realized that there was "dentistry" and then there was "the business of dentistry," and I didn't know a thing about the business of running a dental practice. So I put my office-opening plans on hold and figured I'd better learn something about practice management before I went out and did it all wrong.

They didn't know it at that big practice where I worked, but I spent the next year "apprenticing" myself in the field of the business end of dentistry. I watched everything, and I got real friendly with the ladies who really ran the place, and I asked a lot of questions.

Time out here, while I make a big confession: I am not an original thinker. I really wish that I were, and I have great respect for people who can come up with a new idea; but that's not my strong suit. But I do know a good idea when I see it, and I do have some ability to put good ideas together and to put good ideas and good people together. I got a lot of good ideas while working in that practice and discarded some that I recognized as not so good. But that was the beginning of my 25-year learning experience, and it's still going on. I've been out of dental school for 30 years now, and I'm sad to say that when I run into some of my classmates, I realize they've been practicing just one year–1 year times 30. They're still doing things the way they did the first year out. And they run their practices the way they were taught to in dental school. You remember how they taught you to run your practice in school, don't you?

So I'm an observer and a collector and a sorter and organizer of good ideas, but I'm also an experimenter. I've always been willing to try something out to see if it works. If it does, I've found another good idea. If it doesn't, I'm just as ready to chuck it and move on. By the way, that's a lot harder to do. It's like admitting I was wrong. Maybe that's why so many dentists hold on to ways of doing things and ways of thinking far beyond the point at which they don't work any more. It just seems so hard for most of us to say, "I made a mistake."

By the end of 1965, I figured I had a good enough collection of good ideas and good enough location to open a practice. On the day before I opened my doors, my parents drove over from Baltimore to see the office. After my father had looked around, he gave me a piece of advice that I've never forgotten, that I use every day, and that I believe will be the most useful thing I know in good times and bad. Here's what he said: "Son, I don't know anything about dentistry, but I do know something about business and about people. If you want to be successful, you take good care of people, and they'll take good care of you."

Now I spotted that right away as a really good idea, and one that's worth repeating in capital letters.

TAKE GOOD CARE OF PEOPLE, AND THEY'LL TAKE GOOD CARE OF YOU.

Years later, I saw it put somewhat differently:

"You can get everything you want in life, if you help enough other people get what they want."

Armed with that good advice and the stuff I'd learned in my "apprenticeship," I started practicing, and my preparation paid off well. I was paying the bills from the first week and showing a profit by the third month, and it didn't take me long to figure out that I had it made. I was making more money than I ever dreamed possible, and the numbers just kept going up.

Sometime around 1968, I bought a book by Bob Levoy titled *How to Build the $100,000 Practice.* (Levoy's audio tape series, *The Solid Gold Practice,* is available from PennWell Books). To put things in perspective, the $100,000 practice in 1968 would be the equivalent of the $500,000 or $600,000 practice of today. I thought I was doing pretty well and had grossed $68,000 that year. That book was right up my alley. It was chock-full of good ideas, and I went right to work using them. I can't even remember more than one of them now-something about keeping little plastic rain bonnets handy to give out to ladies so they wouldn't get their bouffant hair-do's messed up. We did that and everything else Levoy suggested, and it worked! By 1970 the practice grossed over $100,000. Unbelievable!

Two years later, 1972, I hit the wall, a really bad case of "burn out." The practice was doing fine, predictably so. It was so predictable, as a matter of fact, that when I looked out at the horizon of my professional career, all I could see was one year following the other each with its predictable 15 percent increase, ad infinitum, on and on, into the future, until I hung up my drill or died. The challenge was over. All the excitement of wondering if I could build a successful practice was over. I'd done it. There had even been a recent article in Dental Economics that confirmed my success. According to my gross income for that year, I was in the top two percent of all the general practices in the country. The top two percent! Terrific! But where do you go from there? From there, it's just "more of the same," and I was bored out of my gourd.

I found the answer to my dilemma in continuing education and rejuvenated my enthusiasm for dentistry with courses in molar endodontics, occlusion, crown and bridge, and implantology.

Learning new skills and sharpening my old ones kept me excited about dentistry for about five or six years, but by the end of the seventies I had gotten pretty slick at it, and the boredom was beginning to creep back in. I started noticing that dentistry was something I had to "get out of the way" each day so I could get on to the things I really wanted to do. Since I was only 45 years old and figured I had at least another 15 professional years ahead of me, that was a rather chilling attitude.

And then I heard about Quest. Now I've got to say that in recent years I've heard a lot of negative comments about Quest. I don't know if they're true or not, but back in 1980 when I signed up to do the full management course with them, I thought they were the best thing that had come along since sliced bread. I was in the sixth group that went through their course, and I think I was the first (or at least one of the first) East Coast dentists to take it. I went out to Reno twice for long weekends and to Dallas twice with my staff. It was expensive to say the least, but our team found a game to play. We found out there was no limit to the kind of practice we could have, no limit to the kind of service and care we could give to our patients.

We came back from that course really fired up and set out to revamp the whole practice. We got rid of an associate who was just taking up an operatory and gave it to the hygienist as a second room. We took all the "administrative" tasks away from her and gave her an assistant to do them. Her assistant was in the room with a hygiene patient going over medical and dental history, taking blood pressure, giving oral hygiene instructions, and taking x-rays; while the hygienist was in the other room with another patient, doing what she went to school to learn to do: scaling and polishing and motivating people to take better care of their mouths. Everybody was a winner. The patients got better, more consistent care, and the hygienist got to do hygiene instead of washing instruments. Up in my three operatories, we were learning how to really use the skills of a well-trained assistant and how to schedule effectively and for optimum dental care. Everybody in the practice got involved in generating patient rapport and in promoting good, complete dentistry.

The word started to get out in the community that we were doing something "special," and our numbers of patient referrals more than doubled. Now we really had a game going! We were good, and we knew it. The game was: Could we provide good quality dentistry in a loving and caring environment for as many people as wanted us to take care of them, and not compromise any of our standards, but continue to upgrade them? That was one hell of a challenge. That was a game that got me up and running every morning, and I loved it! I also didn't mind the increased income that went along with it–nor did the staff, who were taking home some hefty bonuses most months.

By mid-1981, the practice productivity had doubled from 1980, and local dentists were becoming aware that something was going on over at my place. A few of them wanted to come over and have a look, and we let them. But we soon realized that all they saw was a busy office. I told them about Quest, but they were all turned off at the idea of going out to the West coast. That's when I recognized the need for a local program that would teach dental team development and all the management stuff I was using. So I got together with Ken Schatz, the business consultant I had worked with, and we put together a ten-month program called Partners on Purpose. Over the next five years, just about 50 dentists in the Baltimore/Washington area went through our program. I don't want to take all the credit, because most of them were fine practices before we got a hold of them, but our graduates run some of the very best dental offices in our area. And they just keep getting better.

By 1984, I had a staff of nine, and we had taken on a young dentist just out of school to be my "intern". He did all the "scut work" for me, so I could concentrate on doing the important stuff. He gave all the injections, packed and carved amalgams, and took crown and bridge impressions, things like that. As a team we were productive, we did good dentistry, we had a great reputation in the community, and we were having a good time outside the office too. We bowled together and went ice skating and white water rafting. We even took trips together to the Bahamas and Aruba, all paid for by the practice as extra bonuses.

To the dental community around us, we were looking pretty good. Sometimes alone and sometimes as a group we gave talks and presentations to study clubs and dental societies. We had become "experts."

Then in April of 1984, the staff and I went to hear Rick Kushner give his Lean and Mean Seminar. We walked out of there with our heads spinning. That man said things that transformed the whole way we looked at our practice–what we "owed" the public, what they owed us, and what the "bottom line" that really counted was.

As I've said, I usually recognize a good idea when I see one, and this fellow Kushner had a lot of them. What I haven't told you yet is that, as a group, we've learned to overcome the single most devastating barrier to growth and movement-procrastination. We really don't mess around. When we zero in on something we think will be good for the practice, we roll up our sleeves and jump in and get it done. Three weeks after listening to Rick, we had completely revised the financial structure of the practice and were on our way to setting straight what we didn't learn from Quest. One month after the Lean and Mean Seminar, I flew out to Denver and spent a day in Rick Kushner's practice. That trip was invaluable. Rick is a very innovative guy who really knows how to run a dental practice. I'll get into the changes we made as a result of his seminar and my visit later on, but I just want to acknowledge him for the contribution he's made to our practice, and to so many others around the country.

We have gotten "leaner" and "meaner" in the practice. We got rid of our "intern" and are down to a staff of six, and we still get the job done. And we might have to get "leaner" and "meaner," but thanks to Rick Kushner, we know how to do that. So that's how we got to where we are.

Does all of that history make me look like the kind of guy who runs after whatever's "in" or "new" or "the thing to do"? Well, I'm really not, but I do believe that the one constant in life is change. Things do change, and circumstances change, and situations change. And the only way I know how to deal with change is to be observant and watch for it, and then to be flexible enough to go with it, to make it work for me and not against me.

Granted, I'm probably very prejudiced, but I can honestly say that dentists are some of the finest people I know. We are (for the most part) hard-working, conscientious, self-critical (sometimes too much so), and dedicated. We perform intricate and demanding tasks under often difficult and sometimes impossible conditions. We are professionals in the best sense of the word, and in order to survive economically, we must also be good businessmen/women.

That's the area where most of us fall short. And the hard truth is that if you can't keep your practice financially viable, you don't get to deliver the services you're capable of to the public.

Up until now, using good management skills (notice I said using, not knowing) was something we could choose to do if we wanted to be more successful. With the changes that may be coming our way, successful dentists will need to sharpen their management skills, and many of our colleagues who chose to ignore them will have to learn now or face the possibility of going under.

So I'm writing this book as a kind of "pay back," a way of giving back to dentistry something that I have acquired over the years that I believe could be crucial to many of my colleagues. For in the years ahead running a good business may no longer be a "good thing to do": it may very well become the difference between staying in practice or not.

This book, for some of you, will be a checklist; you may finish it, and say, "Well, we're doing all of that," although I certainly hope every reader will come away with enough ideas to justify the time spent reading it. But for some, this could be a "survival manual." In either case, I've tried to put things down in a practical, useful way so that you don't just pick up some good ideas, but that you know how to take them into your practice and put them to work.

Now I've already told you I don't consider myself to be an original thinker. When you do come across an idea in this book that I thought up myself, I promise to take full credit for it. Most of what you read here will probably not be new to you. If you've kept up-to-date on dental practice management over the past five to ten years, you will have heard most (if not all) of what I have to say here, although I've attempted to look at all of it anew in light of what I think we may have to deal with in the years ahead.

So why have I bothered to write all this down, and why am I asking you to read it? Well, I've said I'm no creative thinker, but I am a good organizer (you should see my closet), and I know how to put things together (to mix and match, so to speak). That's what I've set out to do in this book–to take 10 or 15 or 20 years of things I've learned and things I've tried and things I've read, and put them all together in an organized and orderly way so you can use them to get your practice organized and ready for good times, if we're lucky, or difficult times to be in business (practice), if we're not.

Has this material ever been put down on paper before? Of course it has! And I'm sure that if you took the time and trouble, you could dig through your back issues of *Dental Economics* or *Dental Management* or Earl Estep's *Country Gold* or Dr. William Oates' *The Winning Combinations I, II,* and *III* and pull out what you need to know and to do, right now, for your practice. Well, I've done that for you, plus a lot more. I've not only read all that material, I've tested a good deal of it out in my laboratory (practice), and I have a pretty good idea as to what works and what doesn't. It's taken me a long time to do that, and with the tidal wave of change that may be headed our way, you've got no time to reinvent the wheel.

But how do you know that what worked in my laboratory will work in your practice?

For one thing, my practice is about as "average" as you can find. We practice outside a large city, but we're in a rural/suburban area. Our patients run the gamut from low income to a U.S. senator and some members of the House of Representatives. But the majority are white and blue collar families in the lower middle income range. Our fees are, for the most part, right in line with everybody else practicing around us. What works for us, I feel very confident, would work in just about any dental practice I could think of. But I don't make that statement without evidence. All of the things we do have been passed on to the 30 or 40 dentists that I've worked with in the past five or six years. We're all doing basically the same stuff, and it works just as well in a fancy downtown office and in affluent suburbs as it does for us. So I feel very confident in telling you it will work for you. Your job is to put it to work, to go into your practice and do it!

The hardest things for most people to overcome are inertia and procrastination. Most of us need some motivation to get us going. I can't think of a better motivator than the economic changes that every practice has to deal with. So use it to get your practice in the best possible shape. If the economy stays strong and healthy, the worst thing that can happen is that your practice will get better. I actually hope that's the case, but I'm not counting on hope, and you shouldn't either.

CHAPTER ONE

THE SUCCESSFUL PRACTICE OF THE FUTURE

It seems appropriate to begin this chapter with some definition of the word "success." When we hear it said of someone that he is "successful," certainly financial success comes to mind, and a successful dental practice assuredly is fiscally stable. A successful practice should be able to comfortably pay its bills, provide the doctor with a life-style commensurate with the time and effort he has expended in obtaining his education, and assure the doctor an adequate retirement fund. A fiscally stable practice should also have sufficient reserves on hand or available to meet unexpected emergencies, including at the least a short-lived downturn in the economy.

By definition, then, the successful practice should have the ability to thrive in good times, and at least to survive in bad times.

A successful dental practice should also have a reputation in the community it serves that assures the continued growth of the practice, and a sufficient number of new patients to secure its future, both for the doctor as well as for a second generation professional to whom the doctor may choose to transfer the practice.

It has been said that the one constant in life is change. Things do change. Always. And yet, when most of us look into the future of our professional lives, we tend to extrapolate the past and the present into the future. It is indeed difficult to imagine that, in our professional

1

lifetimes, things can become much different than they are right now, but just look behind you: who could have predicted some of the dramatic changes that we've witnessed in the past ten or fifteen or twenty years? The high-speed handpiece was introduced to me, very cautiously, in 1959, when I was a senior in dental school. I was taught to do dentistry standing up and had to relearn everything in order to work from a sitting position. I was taught as a student that people didn't have enough manual dexterity to floss their teeth. Who would have anticipated the revolution that Bob Barkley started when he began teaching effective oral hygiene? Or the effects of fluoridation. Or the amazing increase in dental insurance coverage. Or the onslaught of the capitation plans, the clinics, the HMOs and the PPOs. Or the threat of AIDS. Cosmetic dentistry. Implantology. All are major changes that have shaped our profession and our practices in a relatively short period of time.

Were those changes predictable? Could the astute practitioner of the late fifties have been able to see what lay ahead? I doubt it. And yet, as in any business, shortsightedness in dentistry can be disastrous.

While I don't advocate trying to predict the future, I do believe that the successful dentist, operating in the environment of the 1990s and beyond, must understand the role that change will play on his practice. He or she, in order to remain successful, must be on the constant lookout for change, and maintain a practice posture that is both ready and able to use those changes for continued growth. While the dentist of the fifties and sixties could practically ignore change, and the practitioner of the seventies and eighties had to be only somewhat observant, in today's world success in practice requires intense vigilance, for not only is change a constant, but the rate of change increases with time. Technical as well as economic and social change seems to be coming at us with ever-increasing speed. If success in the past had a certain element of luck attached to it, luck will play less and less of a role in the future. Success will come, and remain, with the professionals who keep current with what is happening in dentistry, as well as in the world around them, and who can use that awareness to continually move their practices ahead.

Within my lifetime, as a patient and dentist, I have been able to watch our profession pass through a number of phases. Most of my observations have been in hindsight, but certainly the dental practice of the 1950s was not the same as the practice of the sixties, and we have all seen the changes that have affected the profession in the last twenty years, giving the practices of the seventies and eighties their uniqueness.

The changes in the way that we practice dentistry today represent an evolution that has been going on since the late 1950s, an evolution which has become predictable and which must be taken into consideration by the young dentist just beginning a practice, as well as by the mid-career practitioner who plans to remain competitive for the next ten to twenty years.

What will the successful practice of the 1990s look like? Certainly, it will be a far cry from the "one girl" or "no girl," single operatory, over-the-drug-store practice that I visited as a boy in the 1950s. Surely, it will be different from the "Golden Age" practices of the 1960s with their luxurious patient to dentist ratios. But it will also look different than the eighties practices, which struggled through the onslaught of the HMOs and PPOs.

Where are the trends taking us, and how must the success-oriented dentist structure his practice in order to flourish in the coming decade? While you may take exception to some of my assumption, this much is clear: The days of the one or two operatory practice, located at the end of the corridor on the fifth floor of an office building and run by an unmotivated, outdated technician, are over. Not that a dentist can't eke out a living in such an environment, or in a home-office location; but they will become the exceptions, and they will struggle to survive, with real success virtually impossible. For the practices of the 1990s and beyond will have to be strong enough and solid enough and aggressive enough to present themselves as a recognizable alternative to the clinics and HMOs and PPOs, and viable enough to resist the insurance industry and the capitation plans. Patients will need to perceive a very clear difference in the kind of care they receive in such a practice, as compared to a clinic, and must be willing to pay for that difference. And I don't mean just dental care. I mean the kind of total caring that today's successful practices have learned to provide, and tomorrow's practices must be in the habit of delivering.

I happen to practice in a small shopping mall that is owned and operated by a local food chain. They have one of their stores in the mall, and about eight years ago, they put in a closed panel dental plan for their employees. The plan covered 100 percent of just about all dental services, but the employees had to go to a plan dentist. That was eight years ago, and in the beginning, they all used the plan. But time has passed, and the store's employees have had enough experience with the closed panel system to find out what it's all about. The majority of them still use the plan, but a lot of the store's employees have become patients of ours. They are willing to pay my full fee to have their dental work done, even though they could go somewhere else and get it for free! And that's what all the practices of the future will have to be able to do–to present themselves as a clear enough alternative to the clinics and closed panels so that enough people will be willing to pay for the difference. And the difference needs to be a very measurable perception, on the part of the patient, as to the kind of care and service and attention he or she receives. If we're not doing anything better or more than the clinics, why in the world should they pay us?

There are places in the country today where 50 percent of the population has available some form of capitation or closed panel dentistry, and the trend is toward more of the same. Does that spell the death of the fee-for-service practice? Perhaps it does for some, but certainly not for all. The practices that learn to take outstanding care of people will always find enough people who are willing to pay for that kind of care. Developing that kind of practice will be the greatest task of the years ahead.

As if that doesn't present a big enough challenge, the practice of the future will, I believe, also need to be financially secure enough to survive some difficult economic times. I am, by no means, a pessimist, but as a realist and a pragmatist, I don't see how we can get through the next decade without paying the economic price for our excesses of the past twenty or thirty years. And, in the next chapter, I will spell out for you the "normal" ups and downs of the economic cycle and also the potentially big "dip" that we may be facing in time. Perhaps we'll be lucky and the "readjustment" for our years of living on borrowed money will be short-lived and relatively painless, but in structuring the successful practice for the 1990s, I've also taken a hard look at what we need to do in order for our practices to deal with hard times.

In examining that particular issue, I've discovered that everything that I know or have read or listened to about dental practice management is based on the assumption that our economy will stay strong and healthy forever. No one has addressed the problem of managing a practice in a down economy, and so, with so many experts forecasting some kind of economic difficulties in the 1990s, I've tried to build into my model some safeguards to blunt the effects of such a possibility.

When I look back over almost thirty years of general practice, I can see very clearly that I've been through the ups and downs of at least four national economic cycles. And, undoubtedly, what's happening in our nation's economy, as well as our local economy, does have an effect on our dental practices.

I've also noticed that as my practice has grown stronger and healthier, it is able to more easily sail through downturns in the economy. Before I had built up a large following of loyal patients, for example, I felt a very direct effect on the practice whenever we had even a mild recession. Today, we are able to get through the minor downturns with hardly a ripple. Before we had the financial part of the practice under control, our accounts receivable would go through the roof whenever there was a slight dip in the economy. Now we are prepared to take a flexible response to credit and collections that will maintain our financial viability, even if the economy should get really bad.

So in laying out the essentials for creating the practice of the nineties and into the next century, you'll notice that I've addressed each area from both points of view: a good economy and a bad one. As you move along, you'll probably notice that a practice that has really developed the basics will also be in the best possible position to deal with hard times economically.

If you'll allow me to be somewhat philosophical, there is a component of success that is seldom addressed directly, but it is such a vital component that I don't know of a successful dentist who doesn't have it. For lack of a better name, I'll call it "the joy of practice."

Do you really understand how incredibly fortunate you are, as a private practice general dentist, to have such total control over your work environment? You have no boss. You do not work in a bureaucratic system. No one tells you what to do or how to do it. You have the potential to organize your working days and hours as you see fit. You can work seven days a week or two. You can take two hours for lunch or no lunch. You can choose to work with people you like (really, you can). Your office can look like an antique shop or a penny arcade.

I can't tell you what your practice should be like, but I can tell you that successful dentists have practices that are an extension of their interests and personalities. I know of a dentist who realized that he was definitely a "night person." He and his wife have no children and live in an apartment above the practice. They love to sleep late and to do things together during the day, so his office hours begin at 4:00 P.M. and go until midnight. He takes a dinner break from eight to nine and goes upstairs to eat with his wife. He has attracted a staff that likes to work when he does. Some of them are working a second job. Do you think he has any trouble filling his appointment book? Not at all. He caters to people whose internal clocks or job schedules work like his. He takes care of a special segment of the population, and he does it his way.

And that's the real beauty of our profession. We are, indeed, one of the last of the free-spirited entrepreneurs. We are truly blessed with the possibility of creating our practices just the way we want them to be. I knew of a young dentist who wanted to set up practice in his small home town in a Georgia farm community. Everybody in town told him the place definitely didn't need another dentist. But he opened up anyway, right over the drug store. Not only did he open his practice in a place where there was obviously no need, but he did something even crazier. He didn't want to be a "pull and fill" country dentist. He wanted to do fine dentistry and complete dentistry, and so he set up his practice so that prospective patients knew from the start that his minimum fee was $2,000 (that was in the early seventies). As you can imagine, folks didn't come beating down his door. He didn't have what we would call a "fast start," but he stuck to his guns and very slowly began to attract the kind of patients he was interested in treating. People who needed, wanted, appreciated and were willing to pay for complete, high-quality dentistry. He still does not have a high volume practice. His minimum fee is now $6,000, but people come from all over his state (and beyond) to his little office over the drug store to receive the kind of dental care he offers. He has built a success for himself that goes beyond the financial rewards. He has those, too, but he has done it "his way."

I would venture to say that if you, as the Supreme Ruler of your practice, set the rule that you would only treat patients in the nude, you might have a long wait, but you would ultimately build a clientele comprised of all nudists. You certainly would not be an instant success, but if you held out, the word would spread, and the kind of people who wanted their dental work done with no clothes on would find their way to your door. You can have it "your way"–and you should have it "your way."

When you think about it, it's actually crazy not to have your practice be just the way you want it to be. And if part of the definition of "success" is the enjoyment of what you do every day, then regardless of the ups and downs of the economy or problems with the lab or the staff or the patients; if you have created for yourself a work environment that pleases you, you win every day, no matter what.

So look at your practice and ask yourself, "Is this place an expression of me and my interests and my personality?" Are you a photographer? Then cover the walls with your prints. Do you collect–whatever? Then display your collection in the reception area. Are you a traveler? Bring back a poster from every trip and have it framed for the office. As a matter of fact, the more your office represents who you are (as a person), the more "attractive" your practice becomes. I mean "attractive" to new patients.

My brother is an optometrist, and his hobby is collecting movie and sports posters from the 1940s, and he displays them in his reception area. He has people stop into his office every day to look at his collection, and a good number of them stay around for glasses.

An orthodontist friend practices near a local art colony and over the years has traded lots of orthodontics for art, so that today his walls are full of the works of area painters-some still lingering in obscurity, but some with regional and even national reputations. My friend has a reputation, too: as a fine orthodontist, and for having a "must see" collection of local art works. He claims that on many days he gets as much enjoyment from showing his collection as he does from his dentistry.

One of the most successful pedodontists I know is a wonderful magician. What a great combination! Show me a child who doesn't love magic! I'm sure that he also does good dentistry, but I wonder how many families get started with him because of the magic show.

What's your "thing"? Is it golf? How about a collection of old clubs with photos of golfing "greats," and framed layouts of the world's most famous courses?

Is it camping? Can you imagine your reception area decorated with camping furniture and the walls covered with wilderness photo murals?

Your patients really do want to know who you are, not just what you do. Every successful dentist I know uses his practice to express who he is. By so doing, he not only adds to his success, but at the same time, he derives the pleasure of working in an environment in which he feels comfortable and happy.

Look around you. Does your practice reflect who you are? It is really a blank canvas, waiting for you to create. As a dentist, one of the last of the solo entrepreneurs, you would be foolish to never pick up the brush, to miss the chance to do your work every day in a place that pleases you and supports you in your professional efforts.

The following nine chapters will lay out for you, in great detail, a game plan for the future. It is actually a road map for success, designed to build a solid practice for the young doctor and to create, for the established practice as well as the new practice, a model that will blunt, as much as possible, the effects of bad economic times. If your practice is basically sound, you may need to do little more than some "fine tuning." If, on the other hand, you finish this book with a long "to do" list, I urge you to act without delay. Some of the recommendations I'll make are easily accomplished, but some are long-term projects that need to be started now in order to be in place when and if hard times come our way. "Waiting to see what happens" could very well postpone action until it's too late. By the time you recognize that your practice is being affected, you won't have the time to take counter measures; and by the time you do, the next wave of change could be upon you. The time to act is now. The time to prepare your practice is right away.

To quote Plato, "Chance favors the prepared mind."

CHAPTER TWO

RIDING THE ROLLER COASTER

I like to think of myself as a curious person with a wide range of interests. When I play Jeopardy! or Trivial Pursuit, I usually do well, because I know at least a little bit about most subjects. But economics is one area that I've consistently stayed away from. It's not that I wasn't interested. It was just that every time I tried to learn something about the topic, I came away more confused than when I started. I came to the conclusion that I just wasn't smart enough to figure out what the economists were talking about. Everyone I tried to read seemed to be saying something different, but they were all using the same "facts" to substantiate their opinions. Then I read the results of a scientific study that made me feel a lot better. Some researcher figured out that if you lined up all the economists in the world, head to toe, they couldn't reach a conclusion.

Even the stock market doesn't make any sense to me. People call their brokers for advice on stocks to buy, and the brokers with great confidence (maybe that's where the term "con" comes from) tell them which ones to invest in that will make them a ton of money. But if stock brokers know so much, how come there aren't many (honest) wealthy stock brokers?

Then there are the "explanations" for why the market went up or down on any given day. They never make any sense to me either. For example: "Prices fell on the New York Stock Exchange today as Wall Street reacted nervously to news that the president had a cancerous growth removed from his nose." Can anyone tell me what the president's nose has to do with the relative value of stocks of American companies? Like I said, maybe I'm just not smart enough to figure out economics.

On October 6, 1987, the stock market took a 91 point fall. Here's how the Wall Street Journal explained it: It was Senator Howell Heflin's announcement that he would vote against Robert Bork's nomination to the Supreme Court.

Another example: Everybody knows that nothing perks up the U.S. economy like a war. Why then is the threat of war, any war, anywhere used to explain why the market went down that day? Seems to me that news of a good lucrative war would send stocks up, not down, but that shows you how much I understand about economics.

Actually, I've come to think about economics the same way I think about gnathologists. They both use words to make relatively understandable information confusing enough so as to justify their positions as "experts."

So, in trying to figure out something about economics, I've intentionally stayed away from the experts. I've looked for understandable explanations, ones that make good common sense to me. Also, being a pragmatist, I've looked for explanations that will lead me to decisions. Decisions that can lead to actions.

I'm not writing this chapter to establish myself as an authority on economics. My only intentions are to try to clear up the smoke screen of misinformation that we've been living with for so long, and to help you appreciate the urgency of organizing your practice to deal with what may lie ahead of us.

No one who knows me would ever call me a pessimist, and my projections for our country's economic future are not those of a "doom and gloomer." This nation is too strong and too powerful to go down the drain. But in the interest of protecting my practice, the source of my income, I need to take a realistic look at how the economy has worked historically, and where we are today, and where we may be headed. As a prudent leader of your practice, you need to do the same, not to make you nervous or upset or paranoid, but so that you will be ready with the proper stance to deal with economic change, of whatever severity.

HOW WE GOT TO WHERE WE ARE

Like just about everything else I can think of, economics is cyclical. Things go up and things go down. Nothing, I repeat, nothing goes up forever. People who chart out economic trends can go back into history and plot out the waves of economic growth, always followed by decline and then a new wave of growth. If we wouldn't have had the crash of 1929, a cup of coffee would probably cost about $35 today, and if we don't have a "major readjustment" soon, that cup of coffee will probably cost $150 by the year 2010.

In those waves of economic history, the up side of each wave is driven by inflation, and the down side is driven by deflation.

Basically, two elements influence the economy: natural economic laws, like supply and demand, and government actions.

Governments are comprised of politicians, and what politicians want is to get reelected. History will show that governments always inflate their currency. When times are bad, they pump money into the economy to get it going and make things better. When things are good, they print more money to keep the "good times" rolling. Either way, the constituents are kept happy, and chances for reelection are good. As the government keeps the inflation going, the public has the illusion of an increased standard of living. And actually, especially at the beginning of an upward cycle, that is the case. But, in order to keep inflation going, the government needs to pump in more and more money, money it doesn't have but has to borrow and pay interest on.

Now businesses and investors know that in times of inflation it's smart to be in debt, to borrow as much as you can with today's dollars and buy something that will have its value driven up by inflation. So "leveraged" investments are the thing to do during an inflationary period.

Psychology also plays a role in how the economy works. People who have been through "bad times" are generally more conservative and cautious than those who have not. That's why most inflationary waves last about 50 years. They are fueled by the optimism of people who have no personal experience of anything but up, up, and more up. At some point, all good common sense goes out the window. People, for example, always believed that they could either have "guns" or "butter," until Lyndon Johnson told them that they could have both. It didn't take the public long to catch on. If the government can have it all and not have to prioritize, why can't they do that in their personal lives?

Credit cards and instant loans have blurred the distinction between assets and borrowing, so people have lost sight of their economic limitations.

We all do have economic limitations, individuals and governments alike. Could you imagine you and your spouse borrowing enough money to support a Donald Trump lifestyle for the rest of your lives? Borrowing enough money that there would be no possible way to repay it in your lifetime, or your children's lifetimes, or their children's lifetimes?

Even if you wanted to, you couldn't do that. The banks wouldn't let you. They do have some limitations as to how far they're willing to go in extending personal credit. But the government doesn't operate under any such restrictions. Remember that governments are made up of politicians, and politicians need to get reelected, and what it takes to get reelected is to keep the "good times" rolling. And the way to keep the "good times" rolling is to pump in more money, even when it doesn't make any logical sense.

By the time the Vietnam War was over, for example, we had run up a hefty tab trying to fight that war (the "guns") and fighting the social war at home (the "butter" of the Great Society). We all go on spending sprees, from time to time, but when the bills come in, we usually sober up and realize it's time to tighten our belts and take care of our debts. That's the prudent thing to do in our personal finances, but governments can't take the risk of not remaining popular with the voters, and nothing turns off voters like a recession or worse. So by the time the bills came in for Lyndon Johnson's "guns" and "butter," we had new people in Washington who had their own reelections to worry about and were certainly not going to ask the American people to tighten their belts to pay off debts that their administration hadn't even run up.

This country's fiscal deficit for 1981 was $55 billion, and the Wall Street Journal lashed out at the Carter administration for its irresponsibility and the fact that it was projecting a $28 billion deficit for 1982. The Journal further noted that the way things are going, "we'd be starting at a budget deficit in fiscal 1982 of a lot closer to $100 billion."

After eight years of "supply-side" economics, with a more than doubling of the public debt to over $2 trillion in that short span, with annual deficits routinely in the hundreds of billions, with a net debt to foreigners that has risen to over half a trillion dollars, a $100 billion deficit would be greeted with great relief.

It's just an economic fact of life that the farther along we are in an inflationary period, the more money it takes to keep it going. Here's why: In the beginning of an inflationary period, most of the debt used to drive it goes into business and industry, which use the money to create goods and services that, in turn, fuel the economy. In the later stages of a cycle of inflation, more and more of the debt goes to pay off the interest on the accumulated debt and into government programs that don't generate any goods or services.

Consider this quote from Lee Iacocca in the March 12, 1990, Newsweek editorial:

"It's tax time again in America, and I've got some bad news for everybody who lives west of the Mississippi: all individual federal-income-tax dollars collected in those states in 1989 will buy absolutely nothing. They will not buy the Army a single bullet or cover the cost of a single food stamp. They won't even help out the new pay raise for Congress. Every dime of your taxes will be needed to pay interest on the national debt for one year. Nothing else. And next year, all your taxes will go to the same place. And the year after that, and the year after that."

He goes on to say that our present national debt is not like any other debt because, realistically, we now have to consider it as permanent. In fact, it's a virtual certainty that the principal will never be paid down. We've created a congenital $3 trillion handicap that will be visited on every generation of Americans to come, a bitter legacy for our kids. Adding even another dollar to it should be considered a form of fiscal child abuse. Up to a point, our budget deficits were simply irresponsible. Now, they're patently immoral. We can no longer get rid of the debt. At best, we can freeze it, but that means no more deficits. We should have no more government than we are willing to pay for with no new debt. But how do we even make that attempt with a political system that sustains itself on a something-for-nothing myth? Right now there's no accountability and no political courage to tackle our debt problem.

Now add to the national debt the enormous cost of the Savings and Loan bail outs and the HUD fiasco, and the burden becomes overwhelming. The debt is just too big.

I hear people say, "We've always had debt, but the government always works it out." But there has never been any debt in recorded financial history that even comes close to the percentage of debt we have today. The debt is just mind boggling. But debts are always paid, eventually, either by the borrower or the lender. As long as the borrower is paying, expanding his business and producing, good times prevail. But when the borrower over-borrows and can no longer pay even the compounding interest on the debt, then the cycle automatically reverses itself. And it's taking more and more economic energy, hidden by the smoke and mirrors of political rhetoric, to keep the ball in the air.

In the short time of 10 years, we've gone from the world's biggest creditor nation to its biggest debtor. For years now we've had a growing trade deficit. More and more of our dollars are in the hands of the Japanese and Germans. They don't find much in our "service economy" to buy from us with those dollars, so they lend them back to us so we can use them to pump up our economy and keep the "good times" rolling, that is, to maintain our national life-style. Our foreign investors know that we're all tied together in an international economy, and they worry that if we go down, they'll go with us. But how much longer they'll be willing to underwrite our inflated life-style is growing questionable. If our interest rates don't stay high enough to attract and hold them, they could easily look elsewhere, and we can't cover our debt without them. The global economy is skating on thin ice.

America is borrowing more than $10 billion per month from the rest of the world to finance its huge trade deficit. With present policies and exchange rates, that deficit will never fall below $100 billion and will probably start rising again soon.

Foreigners could halt their investments at a moment's notice, as they did twice in 1987. They could, in fact, liquidate some of the $1.5 trillion in current dollar holdings. The dollar would plunge. With the economy at full employment, prices would rise sharply. Interest rates would soar, triggering a recession. Our fragile financial system would be severely jarred. And no policy tools would be available to respond, with the budget already in huge deficit and tight money required to check inflation.

Some other dubious distinctions: We rank at the bottom of the industrialized world in terms of academic achievement, but we're spending $328 billion a year on public education. We're paying more than any other nation on earth to educate our children, and we have the least to show for it. We are the most violent, crime-ridden nation in the industrialized world. We're also the biggest user of illegal drugs: We have 5 percent of the world's population, and we're using 50 percent of the world's annual output of cocaine. Nine out of 10 of the largest banks in the world are now Japanese; the 10th one is an American bank, but if you took the Third World loans out of it, it would be insolvent.

To many of us, it's hard to accept that Pittsburgh is no longer the steel capital of the world and that Toyota City, not Detroit, is now the automobile capital of the world. In 1960, we made 75 percent of all cars in the world; today we make 25 percent. In 1974, we developed 70 percent of the world's advanced technology. By 1984, our share was down to 50 percent. By 1994, it will be down to 30 percent. The

Japanese are filing more patents each year in our own patent office than we are.

U.S. savings have plummeted to the lowest levels in 40 years. Americans have been on a huge consumption binge in the 1980s, spending more and saving less. Overall, Americans set aside only 3.3 percent of their after-tax income for savings, compared with 12.4 percent for the West Germans and an astonishing 16.8 percent for the Japanese.

Our nation's infrastructure is in a sad state of neglect and demands a huge commitment in funds for a long-needed upgrade. But the money isn't there, not for our roads and bridges or for our schools and factories.

Down through our nation's history, there have been good times and bad times, and it has usually been clear which was which. The 1980s have been different. The decade started with roaring inflation that reduced paychecks, but turned houses into sources of wealth. It lurched back into double-digit interest rates that cooled inflation for a time, but sent the economy into a recession. Then, almost as abruptly, interest rates eased, the economy went from bust to boom, and the stock market took off on a five-year romp that seemed to have nothing to do with the state of U.S. business and industry.

Why have I burdened you with all this "doom and gloom?" Certainly not to frighten you, upset you, or dishearten you. But as the leader of your practice, it is imperative that you have a realistic appraisal of where we are on the economic roller coaster, and where we are probably headed.

Just as no one really knows what makes the stock market go up or down, our economy, too, is out of control. The economists all give the politicians conflicting advice, and we're all looking to the politicians to do something to fix it all up.

But it doesn't take an economic genius to figure out that we are at the end of an economic cycle of inflation. How close are we to the top? No one really knows. But the overwhelming evidence is that no one can do anything to avert an eventual downturn. How severe will the downturn be? That also is a matter for speculation, but the critical issue is this: As a nation and as businesses and as families and as individuals, we have all been borrowing to keep up a life-style that we really can't afford.

Sooner or later (and it looks like sooner), we'll have to pay up. What that will mean is a national lowering of life-style and expectations. We will all have less money available for discretionary spending. Many of the things and comforts that we've come to take for granted may become no longer affordable. We will be forced to prioritize. If we have only so much to spend and can no longer "put it on plastic," we will have to make choices. We will, and our patients will, too. How that will affect your patients will have a very direct bearing on the health of your practice, and consequently on your own life-style.

The bottom line here is that economics is cyclical, and we've been on the up side of the roller coaster for almost 50 years now, longer than the lifetimes of most dentists practicing today. All the indicators seem to lead to the inevitable conclusion that some form of change is on the way. From past history, we know that when economic changes come, weak businesses are in the greatest jeopardy. The stronger your practice is, the better its chances to survive and even thrive under pressure.

In looking back over 25 years of practice, it is clear to me that my practice, like a young seedling, was most vulnerable to bad economic times in its early years. In the beginning, the slightest dips in the economy were felt almost immediately in the appointment book and the cash flow. As the practice grew in strength, its capacity to withstand changes in the economy steadily improved to what it is today: I feel that it could do well in all but the worst kind of depression. And that's what I want for your practice: the firm confidence that you and your staff have everything under control, that all systems are functioning smoothly, and the practice is on course toward ever-increasing success, so that when the storms come, you are ready. But preparation requires time, and the time to prepare is not when you see the storm clouds on the horizon. The time to put your practice in the best possible shape for riding the economic roller coaster is now.

CHAPTER THREE

PUTTING YOUR PRACTICE ON A FIRM FINANCIAL FOUNDATION

As I mentioned before, it's common knowledge that to take the best advantage of a wave of inflation, borrowing money to make investments is a smart thing to do. During the boom days of the late sixties and seventies, smart investors went into debt to "leverage" their investments. Debt that is working for you is good during times of economic expansion and strong inflation.

On the other hand, during deflationary times, it's best to be out of debt. I'll leave others to advise you regarding application of that economic principle to your personal finances, and I would strongly suggest that you take Greg Stanley's Whitehall Management course. He has a thorough understanding of personal finances and knows all of the foolhardy things most of us have done to try to make money. Everyone I know who has followed his advice is in good financial shape because of him.

As for your practice, I make the following recommendations:

> Set a goal to get your practice out of debt as quickly as possible, and assume new practice debt very reluctantly. If you are planning to expand your facilities or purchase new equipment, I suggest that you reexamine your decision in light of that goal. A new practice will, of course, be burdened with start-up debt, but I

maintain that, in an established practice, upgrades and expansions should be financed by the reserves of the practice. With that approach, investments in the future of the practice are paid for by past success, not with hope in the future. If you do decide to go ahead, look to pay cash. If that's not feasible, try to pay off new debt as quickly as possible.

If you have outstanding loans, they also should be paid off as quickly as possible. Get your practice debt free. And the best place to look for funds to reduce or eliminate practice debt is in your accounts receivable.

I want to present you with a system of credit and collections that will dramatically reduce your accounts receivable and leave you with near 100 percent collectable accounts. The system will "clean up" your current accounts, organize your credit extensions, and streamline collections. It also will bring an immediate influx of cash into the practice, which can be used to pay off any existing debt.

BUT FIRST SOME BACKGROUND:

Unless your dental school was different than mine, you left there with the notion that if you went out and took care of the dental ills of the world, you would somehow be financially rewarded. Actually, money, fees, collections, or anything having to do with the "business" of dentistry was never discussed while I was a student. We did, as seniors, have a series of four or five lectures about "practice management" that, even then, I recognized as totally worthless. They were given by a faculty member who had failed in private practice. I understand that things are better now, but probably not much better.

When it came to the financial side of dentistry, here's what I knew: We do the dental work. At the end of the month, we send the patient a bill. They patient sends us the money. If after some amount of time (60 days or 90 days?) he hasn't paid, we send out another bill with a yellow sticker on it. The sticker says: "Have you overlooked this bill? Please be a nice person and send us the money now." If that sticker doesn't produce any results, we go to the blue one, which says: "We haven't heard from you in a long time. This account is really, really past due. Please pay us right away, no fooling!" Now I can't imagine why or how some patients could disregard that blue sticker, but if they do, at the next monthly billing, they get a red one. The red stickers are tough. They say: "If you don't pay this account now, I'm going to tell my lawyer!" Very often the red one gets some action–like a ten dollar check on a $235 balance. But, we say, at least they're paying on the account, and as long as people are paying on their accounts, we can't bother them with any more stickers. If a patient does have the audacity to ignore the red sticker (I never understood how they could) we "turn them over" to a collection agency.

Once a year, we went through the accounts and "wrote off" the bad ones. I never kept track of how much we wrote off over the years, but maybe it's better that way. I think it would be bad for my health to know how much dentistry I've given away in 24 years. In spite of the "weeding out" process, our accounts receivable grew every year. I attributed that to the fact that our gross production was going up as well. With hindsight, I see that's what kept us going. As long as we increased the production, we could pay our bills, but I could never quite figure out why my income hardly went up from year to year.

Those were the "bad" accounts. Then there were what we thought of as basically "good" accounts. We had families (way too many of them) who always had a balance with us. The average was two or three or four hundred dollars. When we sent out our monthly statement, they always paid "something" on the account. So, technically, they were never in arrears. They never even got a yellow sticker, but a typical account looked like this:

> The Smith family had a balance of $285 in January, and we sent them a bill for that amount. They immediately sent back a payment of $75, leaving a balance of $210. In February, two family members came in for checkups, so the February statement announced that they owed us $290. We got back a check for $50, bringing the balance to $240. In March, we got another $50 check, which brought the balance down to $190. In April, Mr. Smith fractured off an upper central incisor and needed a crown, so the statement for that month was for $630. In May, we received a check for $150 that brought the balance down to $480. And so it went with the Smiths, month by month, always a balance and always a payment, but the fact was that they always owed us money. In reality, the Smiths had an interest free loan with us for years.

I mentioned in the Introduction that the practice had taken the Quest Management Seminar in 1981, and that we had learned a great deal from them. Now I'll tell you what we didn't learn. The general philosophy that we heard from Quest was produce, produce, produce. Do whatever you have to do to produce more dentistry. That's the name of the game. If you need more equipment, buy it. If you need more space, rent it or build it. If you need more people, hire them. Just increase the productivity, and everything else will take care of itself. When some of us complained about our rising costs of doing business and increasing accounts receivable, the answer always was, "That's just a symptom of the start up of an accelerated practice. It'll all even out in time."

My accountant didn't much like that answer, but compared to the other dentists he had as clients, my "numbers" were so impressive that he didn't put up much of an argument. After all, we were paying our bills, and my income had almost doubled in two years. So what if it was a smaller percentage of the gross collections? So what if that gross had dropped to 85 percent of the dental work we were producing?

So, while my merry staff and I were busily producing more dentistry than we ever thought possible, what nobody was paying much attention to or cared much about was that our accounts receivable had reached a staggering $150,000 (too much of it uncollectible) and that the bottom line net profit of the practice had dropped into the 20-some percentage range.

Then, in April of 1984, the staff and I attended Rick Kushner's Lean and Mean Seminar. If you haven't done that yet, I strongly urge you to do so. He is a dynamic speaker with a clear sense of the fundamentals of running a business. Rick really turned us around 180 degrees as far as the financial aspect of the practice goes. Before our staff meeting two days later, we had all had a chance to digest what we had heard. All of the staff had realized that there were no other professional services that they used where it was possible to get past the front desk with a "Send me a bill." Neither the optometrist nor the gynecologist nor the veterinarian would let a patient get away with that. Why do dentists still promote the "put it on my tab" mentality? As far as I could tell, there were two explanations. First, there was "tradition." That was just the way things were always done. If it worked in the past, why not in the future? And besides, patients were used to it. It would be shocking to change the system on them. But second (or perhaps really first), we are scared to death that if we ask patients to pay us for the services we render, they might be offended and go somewhere else.

Think about that for a moment. We provide a service or treatment that the patient wants, and from that point on, the burden of being paid for that service is on us; and if we push too hard or are too insistent, they become angry with us and take their business elsewhere. And we worry about losing "good customers" like that! No other business could possibly survive with that attitude.

Speaking of attitudes, have you noticed that your relationship with patients who owe you money is different from your relationship with those who don't? I wasn't able to appreciate that until we had the finances of the practice straightened out. But now, in retrospect, I can explain why some patients were so non-communicative. Now I understand that many of them knew ahead of time that they were not going to pay me. They were allowing me to do their dental work, and they had no intention of paying for it. Knowing that, they didn't want to get too friendly with this guy they were about to cheat so they kept a stand-offish attitude. It's more difficult to rip off someone you've gotten to know and to like.

There was also the strain in the relationships with people who had a "running" balance with us. Maybe we hadn't identified the game they were playing with us, but they knew, and it had to create an uneasiness that brought with them to their visits.

PEOPLE DON'T LIKE PEOPLE THEY OWE MONEY TO.

All of that is gone now, but I could only see and feel it once our financial arrangements with our patients were cleaned up. It's one of those things that only becomes obvious by its absence-like the pain of banging your head against the wall!

Rick Kushner made two statements early on in his seminar, that are crucial to understanding the changes we've made in our financial structure.

> As professionals, we are obligated to the public we
> serve to:
> • Eliminate Pain and Acute Embarrassment.
> • All Other Dental Procedures are Elective.

I suggest that you put this book down for a moment and really think about those two statements.

As professionals we do have an obligation to the public, but what exactly is it? Are we obligated to restore every mutilated dentition to the best of our ability? Are we obligated to replace every missing tooth? To crown every fractured molar? To improve every smile? Obviously not. What then is our obligation? Kushner says, and I agree, that we are obligated to alleviate pain and acute embarrassment. All other dental procedures are elective. That means the patient gets to choose whether or not he or she wants them. They are not needs. People don't need the rest of our services. They may desire them. They may believe they are nice or good to have, but they don't need to have them. The elimination of pain and acute embarrassment aside, everything else we have to offer the public are services that they decide they would like to have, just as they decide to purchase a new TV or take a trip or buy a new suit of clothes.

If you have a problem with those two statements, you will have a problem with the financial arrangements I'm about to suggest, so be sure that we are in agreement. If you are having a problem accepting those statements, I feel very safe in assuming that your accounts receivable are probably out of control, that you are doing a lot of free dentistry, and that you are struggling to pay your bills. (By the way, I do my share of free dentistry, but I get to choose who I'm going to do it for. In the past, the patients got to choose.)

After a thorough discussion of the two statements, my staff and I agreed that, for us, they were true. Based upon our recognition that they were the truth, we instituted the following financial policies, and we put them into effect on the following Monday. (We only waited the two days to give us time to get organized for the changes.)

We are ready and willing to alleviate pain or acute embarrassment for anyone without a financial agreement.

This is the obligation I feel that I owe the public I serve. I would, of course, like to be paid for those services, but if, for whatever reason, the patient cannot pay, I consider that my gift to him or her is my professional obligation.

ALL SERVICES $300 OR UNDER
MUST BE PAID FOR ON THE DAY THEY ARE PERFORMED.

All patients are informed when they make an appointment exactly what will be done at that visit and the fee for those services. They may make payment by cash, check, or credit card. New patients to the practice are told that their first visit will consist of a full series of x-rays, and examination and consultation with the doctor. They are also informed of the fee and told that payment is expected at each appointment.

For services more than $300 there are two options: The patient may pay the fee in full and take a 6 percent discount, or may elect to divide the fee into monthly payments.

Considering the costs involved in billing and collecting accounts, I'm

---

MORTON M. EHUDIN, DDS, PA

9500 LIVINGSTON ROAD
FORT WASHINGTON, MARYLAND 20744
301 248-2020

PATIENT FINANCIAL UNDERSTANDING FORM

Patient Name
and Address:

Parent/Guardian:

Services Performed
Or To Be Performed:

Date Of Services

Fee For Services $_____
Amount Payable By Insurance Plan $_____
Balance Due $_____

The patient (guardian) agrees to be and hereby is fully responsible for total payment to (dentist named above) for procedures
performed in this office including any amounts which are not
covered by dental insurance or prepayment program. If this account should become delinquent at any time, balance in full will
be due upon our request.

I, the undersigned, hereby agree in the event of default in the
payment of any amount due, to pay an additional charge equal to
the cost of collection including agency and attorney fees and
court cost incurred as permitted by the laws governing these
transactions.

The terms of this agreement are as follows:

_____
                    Applicant

_____
                    Witness

Fig. 3–1 Financial Understanding Form

willing to give a patient a discount for cash. Patients who choose to
pay for the services over time are encouraged to make three payments,
although we are willing to go to six payments and occasionally to nine.
They sign a financial agreement with us (Fig. 3–1), and are given a
coupon book (available at any office supply store) for the payments.

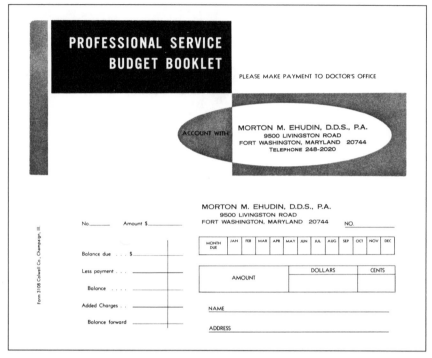

Fig. 3–2 Payment Booklet

Each coupon states the amount of the payment and the exact due date (Fig. 3–2). No major work is begun without a financial arrangement with the patient.

We no longer send out monthly statements.

There is no longer any need to send out statements. Patients who owe us money fall into two categories: Those who have a financial arrangement, have their coupon books, and need no monthly statement, and those whose insurance companies have not yet paid their balance. Patients with dental insurance are expected to pay the uncovered portion of their fees at the time the service is delivered. We will file the insurance forms for them and await payment. If we have not received payment within 45 days after filing, the balance becomes the patient's responsibility. If we are unsure of the percent of coverage, we estimate and make any necessary adjustments when the claim has been paid. For large cases, we are willing to make coupon arrangements for patients to pay their uncovered part of the fee.

Those policies were mimeographed and handed out at the front desk, and were also printed on a poster in the reception area. We were amazed that no one seemed surprised or upset. Really, no one! It appeared as if the general reaction was: "Well, it looks like Dr. Ehudin finally caught on. Too bad, but it was good while it lasted."

Our new policy had an additional benefit: all of the time, energy, and expense involved in getting out the monthly bills was gone for good.

The conversion from monthly statements to coupon arrangements was followed in 1988 by a further refinement, which has taken us completely out of the collection business. Rather than offer patients a coupon arrangement for work over $300, we now offer a dental credit card service. The patient's application is processed through a designated line to our office within 20 minutes. Once accepted, he owes the money to the credit card company, not to us, and we get paid immediately. Why anyone would want one more credit card is a mystery to me, but we have been astounded to discover that most people who live their lives on credit are uninterested in their total accumulated debt. If they want something, their primary concern seems to be finding a way to charge it. The wisdom of that philosophy aside, conversion to the charge cards has even relieved us of the task of tracking coupon arrangements.

That's how we handled the hemorrhage at the front end of the practice. Here's how we cleaned up the accounts receivable. Any patient who had an outstanding balance with us received a letter (see Fig. 3–1), along with the last monthly statement we ever sent out.

I will admit that we sent the letter out and held our breath in anticipation of the reaction. What came back was a flood of money!

When we sent out the letter, our receivables were almost $150,000. We collected more than $75,000 by the deadline date; put another $35,000 on coupon payments, which brought that money in over the next three to six months; identified about $30,000 in insurance; and turned over about $7,000 to a very aggressive attorney for collection. Over the next two years, he managed to collect about $4,000 of that, and we got half.

Today, our receivables are usually around $40 to $50,000. Of that, about $30,000 is insurance, and the balance is all coupon payments.

Here's what we've learned and applied to the area of collections:

- People who are honest and intend to pay their bills will pay them or let you know why they can't.
- Payment arrangements need to be specific ($74 due on April 12).

MORTON M. EHUDIN, DDS, PA

9500 LIVINGSTON ROAD
FORT WASHINGTON, MARYLAND 20744
301 248-2020

Dear Patient,

In a recent meeting with our accountant, we examined the ever-increasing costs of running the practice. He presented us with two alternatives. One was a 10 percent increase in fees, and the second was to discontinue the costly process of monthly billings. In our ongoing efforts to hold down the cost of dental care to all our patients, we have elected the second option.

THIS WILL BE THE LAST MONTHLY STATEMENT YOU RECEIVE FROM THIS OFFICE.

Those patients who have balances with us that are uncovered by dental insurance may choose one of the following options:

DEDUCT 6 PERCENT FROM YOUR BALANCE AND SEND US A CHECK FOR THE REMAINDER IN FULL BY _____.

OR

CALL THE OFFICE-ASK TO SPEAK TO LYNNE-AND MAKE AN ARRANGEMENT WITH HER TO CONVERT YOUR BALANCE TO A MONTHLY COUPON PAYMENT.

For all future services rendered:

PAYMENT FOR SERVICES LESS THAN $300 WILL BE DUE ON THE DAY THEY ARE RENDERED-PAYABLE BY CASH, CHECK, OR CREDIT CARD.

FOR SERVICES MORE THAN $300 YOU MAY ELECT TO PAY IN FULL ON THE DAY THE SERVICE IS RENDERED AND TAKE A 6 PERCENT DISCOUNT, OR YOU MAY MAKE ARRANGEMENTS TO PAY THE FEE WITH A MONTHLY COUPON.

We sincerely appreciate your cooperation in helping us to control the rising cost of dental care. If our new policy causes you problems or inconvenience, please let us know. We are here to serve you.

Many Thanks,

Dr. Ehudin

Fig. 3–3 Outstanding Balance Form Letter

- Payments not made need to be followed up on immediately. We give a five-day grace period and then call to find out where the payment is. Coupon payments are easily tracked through a dated card file.
- If a coupon payment is late, the next payment is nevertheless expected on time.

• If no payment is received by the time the next payment is due, the account is turned over for collection. We, at that point, turn over for collection the entire balance of the account, which then becomes due in full.

The bottom line on credit and collections is that I don't know of one patient we lost because of the change; our practice is on a firm financial foundation; our relationships with patients are clear and clean; and I sleep a lot better at night, knowing that when I sit down to do some dentistry, the odds are very, very good that I'll be paid for it.

I've been recommending this system of credit and collections for over five years now, and I don't know of a single practitioner who has adopted it and isn't delighted. Yet I also find many dentists who consider the possibility and then get cold feet. I think they know that it would work for them, but they also know that once they've committed their practice to that policy, they can't make any exceptions– and what about Mrs. Gotrocks? And then the fear of offending one or some of their patients makes them back off.

Here's how I feel about office policies: They are an expression of your own self worth. If, for example, you have no clear-cut, enforceable policy regarding failed appointments or habitual latecomers, you are sending a very definite message to your patients that your time is not valuable. If you always take the chronically late patient, no matter when he or she comes, the message is that it doesn't matter to you. Why not try on one more outfit? Dr. Milktoast won't mind if I'm late. He always takes me anyway. Why not decide to play another set? "Good old Doc" will just make me another appointment for next week.

Unless you send your patients the unmistakable message that you intend to be paid for the services you provide–and paid in a timely fashion–you make a clear statement about the worth that you place on the work you do. You are saying either that it really isn't worth the fee you're asking, or you really don't need the money, at least not right now.

Your office policies are all a part of the reputation your practice has in your community (Figs. 3–4 and 3–5). Are you satisfied with the reputation that you really don't care if patients show up or not, or show up on time or not, or pay you or not? The word does get around. People do know about your practice, and you will attract a certain following, accordingly. If you are known to be an easy touch, you'll find yourself dealing with a lot of people who are very ready and willing to take advantage of you,

---

MORTON M. EHUDIN, DDS, PA

9500 LIVINGSTON ROAD
FORT WASHINGTON, MARYLAND 20744
301 248-2020

Welcome,

We would like to take this opportunity to thank you for choosing us as your new dentist and to welcome you to our practice.

In order to familiarize you with our office and help make your first visit go smoothly, please take a few minutes to read the rest of this letter and fill out the questionnaire being given to you.

THANKS!!

The purpose of our practice is to provide a safe, friendly, cooperative environment in which our patients can receive quality dental care at a reasonable cost.

It is the intention of everyone who works in this office to see that you receive the very best dental care with as little inconvenience and discomfort as possible. Most people feel some degree of anxiety about having dental work, so we make every effort to see that your visits with us are as easy as they can be. We think that you'll agree with the great majority of our patients that having dental work done at our office "is no more traumatic than having a haircut."

We are aware that good dentistry is not inexpensive. We also know that the best way to keep our patients' dental bills to a minimum is to prevent problems rather than treat them. For adults, avoiding gum disease is our number one concern. Experience has proven that patients who follow a reasonable home care routine and have a cleaning and examination twice a year rarely run into major dental problems. Our goal is to get you into the best dental condition possible, and then maintain that level of dental health through an ongoing program of preventive dentistry.
At your first appointment, unless it is for emergency treatment, all adults will receive a complete oral examination, a series of full mouth x-rays and a consultation. For children/young adults under age 21 we will provide an examination, cleaning, fluoride and bite-wing x-rays.

After your examination, the doctor will discuss any findings with you, make a treatment recommendation and let you know the cost and number of appointments you'll need. Services may be paid for by check, cash, Mastercard, Visa or American Express. If you would like to make special payment arrangements, please let us know in advance and we will be happy to work with you.

Fig. 3–4 Office Policies (New Patient)

and they'll send you their like-minded friends. It's really up to you.

HOW WILL OUR CREDIT AND COLLECTION POLICY BE AFFECTED BY A DOWN ECONOMY?

My assumption is that during hard economic times, more patients will be in need of credit, and collections could become a major

MORTON M. EHUDIN, DDS, PA

9500 Livingston Road
Fort Washington, Maryland 20744
301 248-2020

As a courtesy to our patients with dental insurance, we provide
the following services-if you provide us with the necessary claim
forms and policy information.

We will estimate what your insurance will pay (our "best guess"
based on experience and information provided by you). We will
file your insurance claim for you and wait 45 days for your
insurance carrier to reimburse us. Any amount estimated not to
be covered by your insurance is due as services are rendered.
Any outstanding amounts not paid by insurance will be due
immediately upon billing. If your insurance company has not paid
us in 45 days, we will bill you directly and you will have to ask
your insurance company to reimburse you.

Unlike many professional offices, we pride ourselves on
punctuality. You'll probably notice that (barring unscheduled
emergencies) if we don't see you right at your appointed time,
you'll rarely have to wait more than 5 to 10 minutes. We work
hard to see that we don't keep our patients waiting, but we need
your cooperation. Please keep us on schedule by being on time
for your appointment.

As a courtesy, we will try to contact you the day before your
appointment to remind you. However, it is your responsibility to
keep appointments that you schedule with us. If you cannot keep
a scheduled appointment, please give us at least 48 hours
notification (weekends and holidays excluded). Your appointment
is being reserved especially for you and late cancellations or
failed appointments may mean that a patient who needs that time
may not get to be seen. If we are unable to fill your reserved
time, or have no opportunity to do so, there will be an
appropriate charge for our lost time.

ATTENTION PARENTS!

When you bring in your children (age 18 or under) for an
appointment, we do require that a parent remain in the office at
all times. We understand the temptation to drop them off and get
in some shopping, however, if a situation arises where the doctor
needs to speak to you or get your consent to continue with
treatment we can't go looking for you. Please understand.
If at any time you have any questions about your treatment, fees,
or services, please let us know.

Fig. 3-4 *(Continued)*

problem. Before being called upon to extend more credit to patients,
I would want to be certain that the receivables currently on the books
are "good." It would seem disastrous to me to add new receivables
on top of bad or shaky debt. Also, if we are asked to extend more
credit than we normally do, I want to be certain that we have a system
in place for orderly and monitored collection.

MORTON M. EHUDIN, DDS, PA

9500 LIVINGSTON ROAD
FORT WASHINGTON, MARYLAND 20744
301 248-2020

FAMILY VS. INDIVIDUAL ACCOUNTS

If you would like us to bill you as a family we will do so. The
person who must sign below will be responsible for the entire
account. You may not choose to have your account put in another
family member's name without written consent from that person.

If you prefer, we can bill you individually.

Please check your preference.

☐ Family Account
☐ Individual Account   Signature _____

We provide you with the above information in order to avoid
confusion and misunderstandings. If at any time you are
uncertain about our office policies, please feel free to discuss
them with any of our administrative staff.

I have read and understand the above office policies.

Signature _____ Date _____

Fig. 3–4 *(Continued)*

    If patients lose dental insurance as a benefit, they'll be paying more for dental care than they're accustomed to at a time when money is scarce. A practice without a good system which deals with increased demands for credit will find itself in deep trouble.

    I remember that during the late 1960s, for some reason, engineers in large numbers were out of work. I had half a dozen families who

MORTON M. EHUDIN, DDS, PA

9500 LIVINGSTON ROAD
FORT WASHINGTON, MARYLAND 20744
301 248-2020

Dear Patient:

On the 25th anniversary of our practice, we would like to take a
moment to renew our relationship with you. Please take a moment
to update yourself on the following office policies.

THANKS!!!!

**The purpose of our practice is to provide a safe, friendly,
cooperative environment in which our patients can receive quality
dental care at a reasonable cost.**

It is the intention of everyone who works in this office to see
that you receive the very best dental care with as little
inconvenience and discomfort as possible. Most people feel some
degree of anxiety about having dental work so we make every
effort to see that your visits with us are as easy as they can
be. We hope that you've come to agree with the great majority of
our patients that having dental work done at our office "is no
more traumatic than having a haircut."

We are aware that good dentistry is not inexpensive. We also
know that the best way to keep our patients' dental bills to a
minimum is to prevent problems rather than treat them. For
adults, avoiding gum disease is our number one concern.
Experience has proven that patients who follow a reasonable home
care routine and have a cleaning and examination twice a year
rarely run into major dental problems. Our goal is to get you
into the best dental condition possible, and then maintain that
level of dental health through an ongoing program of preventive
dentistry.

Unlike many professional offices, we pride ourselves on
punctuality. You've probably noticed that (barring unscheduled
emergencies) if we don't see you right at your appointed time,
you rarely have to wait more than 5-10 minutes. We work hard to
see that we don't keep our patients waiting, but we need your
cooperation. Please keep us on schedule by being on time for
your appointments.

As a courtesy, we try to contact you the day before your
appointment to remind you. However, it is your responsibility to
keep appointments that you schedule with us. If you cannot keep

Fig. 3–5 Office Policies Review (Old Patient)

suddenly had no income, but they were all good people, and I was
certain that when the money was available, I would get paid. I sent
them all a letter insisting that they at least keep up their routine exams
and prophys. We never sent them a bill, but just kept a running tab
going and asked them to let us know when they were able to begin
paying on their accounts. I didn't lose a penny on any of them, kept

MORTON M. EHUDIN, DDS, PA

9500 Livingston Road
Fort Washington, Maryland 20744
301 248-2020

a scheduled appointment, please give us at least 48 hours
notification (weekends and holidays excluded). Your appointment
time is being reserved especially for you and late cancellations
or failed appointments may mean that a patient who is in need of
that time may not get to be seen. If we are unable to fill your
reserved time, or have no opportunity to do so, there will be an
appropriate charge for our lost time.

Payment is due as services are rendered. Treatment may be paid
for by check, cash, MasterCard, Visa, or American Express. If
you would like to make special payment arrangements, please let
us know in advance and we will be happy to work with you.
As a courtesy to our patients with dental insurance we provide
the following services-if you provide us with the necessary claim
forms and policy information.

We will estimate what your insurance will pay (our "best guess"
based on experience and information provided by you). We will
file your insurance claim for you and wait 45 days for your
insurance carrier to reimburse us. Any amount estimated not to
be covered by your insurance is due as services are rendered.
Any outstanding amounts not paid by insurance will be due
immediately upon billing. If your insurance company has not paid
us in 45 days, we will bill you directly and you will have to ask
your insurance company to reimburse you directly.
If you have double insurance carrier, we accept payment from the
primary carrier only. You will have to pay the difference and be
directly reimbursed by the second carrier.

ATTENTION PARENTS!

When you bring in your children (age 18 or under) for an
appointment, we do require that a parent remain in the office at
all times. We understand the temptation to drop them off and get
in some shopping, however, if a situation arises where the doctor
needs to speak with you or get your consent to continue with
treatment we can't go looking for you. Please understand.
If at any time you have any questions about your treatment, fees,
or services, please let us know. You can count on us to make
every effort to avoid a misunderstanding, to keep our agreements
with you, and to preserve our friendship.

Fig. 3-5 *(Continued)*

them as patients, and developed a loyalty that has brought innumerable referrals to the practice. In hard times, we may have to take some chances like that. The key to that kind of credit extension is to evaluate the patient's intention to eventually pay, and have a clear agreement with him or her so that there are no misunderstandings. Sending people like that a monthly statement would be a waste of time and

---

MORTON M. EHUDIN, DDS, PA

9500 LIVINGSTON ROAD
FORT WASHINGTON, MARYLAND 20744
301 248-2020

FOR OUR RECORD PLEASE FILL OUT THE FOLLOWING INFORMATION

FAMILY VS. INDIVIDUAL ACCOUNTS

If you would like us to bill you as a family to minimize
confusion and paperwork we will do so. The person who signs for
the family account will be responsible for the entire account.
If you choose a family account please list the names of the
family members who are to be included on the account. You may
not choose to have your account put in another family member's
name without written consent from that individual.

Please check your preference for account billing and list
appropriate names to be attached to this account.

☐ Family Account _____

                  _____

                  _____

                  _____

                  _____

☐ Individual Account _____

Signature: _____ Date: _____

I have read and understand office policies that have been
provided to me.

Signature: _____ Date: _____

Fig. 3–5 *(Continued)*

money, and would only create embarrassment or humiliation.

Flexibility and common sense, coupled with a good system, will be vital to the economic well-being of a practice. Some patients, for example, may need more time to finance work than we are accustomed to giving. Based on our experience with those patients, we have to be ready to accommodate and allow for smaller payments over a longer time frame. This is only feasible if a system is already in place to handle credit properly.

When it comes to collecting delinquent accounts, it may become necessary to use great sensitivity in differentiating between patients who have intentionally taken advantage of us and good patients in financial trouble. Before making rash decisions about turning accounts over for collection, I foresee staff members doing telephone counseling with delinquents to make that determination. That kind of caring can make the difference between futile attempts to collect the uncollectible, and preserving relations with patients of good will and no money. When times return to normal, those people will be eternally grateful.

SUMMARY

In good times, we should be paid for the dentistry we do. In bad times, we must. A practice that has its house in order concerning credit and collections will be best prepared to cope with the changing and challenging times ahead.

BUDGETING FOR A PREDICTABLE INCOME

Several years ago, the management study group that I belong to invited an accountant to talk to us about profitability. Early in the evening, he happened to ask a question, the response to which shocked him. He asked if there were any practices in the group that did not have a fiscal budget. To his amazement, every hand in the room went up-and those were some of the best-run dental practices in our area! When he explained that he didn't know of a small business that didn't have a budget and couldn't understand how we could possible conduct our affairs without one, we invited him back to show us how to develop and use a budget.

Any of us interested in properly managing his or her practice is certainly aware of the averages for various expenses for a general dental practice, for example, 5 percent for rent. But until I understood how to use a budget, that was just historical information. I could look at my numbers at the end of any period and say, "We're staying within the averages," or not. And whether we were close to the averages or not was a matter of pure chance. It was all "after the fact." Those averages are "interesting," but they're not useful. A budget, on the other hand, is a useful tool in controlling the expenses of running a practice.

In creating our practice budget, we had to decide which items to monitor. We quickly realized that we didn't want to use the same items that our accountant monitored. Many of those were constants, like rent, over which we had no control. An item like depreciation also has no place in a budget. Here are the items we chose to include in our budget. In developing your own, you may choose different items. The important thing is that you monitor items over which you and your staff can exercise some degree of control.

Salaries .... includes all salaries other than temporary help.

Bonuses .... includes incentive and Christmas bonuses.

Temporary Help .... expenditures for fill-ins, usually hygienists during vacation time or illness.

Dental Supplies

Lab

Utilities and

Repairs .... budgeting "rent" makes no sense, since it is fixed but these items can be controlled.

Marketing .... includes all external promotional items.

Patient Relations .... includes expenses for newsletters, and in-office give aways (flowers, toys, toothbrushes, etc.)

Office Supplies .... all paper supplies and business office materials.

Professional

Development .... includes continuing education and training.

Professional Fees .... accounting and legal services.

Insurance .... malpractice, business, and medical.

Telephone

Entertainment

Once we had determined what to monitor, we needed some numbers to work with. National averages and percentages didn't seem to be too useful, so we used our own history. We went back over the past three years and came up with the average annual dollar expenditure for each item. Dividing that by twelve, we arrived at a monthly target figure. Then we looked at that figure and asked if we could realistically reduce it. That gave us a "game" to play in each category.

Here's an example, using "Office Supplies," to illustrate how we arrived at a monthly target:

For the three previous years we spent $8,804, $9,316, and $8,270 on office supplies. The total expenditure was $26,390, which averaged out to $8,796. Dividing by 12, we got a monthly target of $733. We then looked at the $8,796 figure and decided that we realistically could cut our costs in that category by $796, so we set an annual goal of $8,000 for office supplies, and a monthly target of $666. That meant we had to look for ways to save $66 a month in office supplies, and that's when the creative part of budgeting comes in. (Fig. 3–6)

The first year that we began using a budget was the most creative, perhaps because there was so much room for cost cutting. Over the years we've gotten to be rather "lean," and without going to ridiculous extremes, there doesn't seem to be much left to cut. But if times get tough, we're ready to look at the "ridiculous" possibilities.

Some of the things we've done to cut office supply expenses, by way of example, are:

- Having a pharmaceutical company print our pre-scription pads instead of paying to have them done.
- Cutting up outdated forms and old stationary to use as scrap paper instead of buying memo pads.
- Using our "old-style" patient charts for emergency patients, until we knew if they would become patients of the practice.

BUDGET FORM								
EXPENSES	JAN	+/–	FEB	+/–	MAR	+/–	APR	
ITEM (MONTHLY TARGET)	Amount Spent							
	Amount Spent Year-to-Date	•						
Dental Supplies (645)	584		590		628		714	
	584	–	1174	–	1802	–	2510	
Office Supplies (505)	572		514		396		428	
	572	+	1086	+	1482	–	1930	
Marketing (250)	0		535		185		410	
	0	–	535	+	720	–	1130	

Fig. 3–6 Budget Form

- Making some of our own "business forms" on the copy machine, instead of buying them.
- Combining our business card and appointment card into one card, and saving printing costs.
- Getting a postage meter instead of buying stamps.
- Eliminating an outdated "patient attitude" questionnaire.
- Putting old (over five years) full series periapical x-rays into envelopes so we could reuse the x-ray mounts, instead of buying new ones.
- Finding a cheaper envelope to mail out full sets of x-rays.

Those were just some of the things we did to control our costs in just one area of the practice, but it really paid off. Our total expense for office supplies in the first year of budgeting was $7,783. That was $217 under budget, a savings of $1,013 compared to the average for the preceding three years. We had been spending at a rate of $733 per month. We targeted to bring that down to $666, and we actually reduced it to $648.

Obviously, we weren't able to do that in every category. In some, we just managed to stay on target. In a few, we went over budget. But for the year, we managed to reduce our costs by more than $8,000.

Here are some rules of budgeting that we've discovered:

- The numbers need to be reviewed every month. Without that kind of close scrutiny, too much time goes by to take any corrective action.
- No cost-cutting action can affect the quality of the care we provide. (There are offices, for example, that use cloth towels instead of paper towels to cut costs.)
- Everyone needs to be involved in planning cost cuts.
- Everyone needs to be kept up-to-date as to how we're doing.
- Everyone needs to share in the savings.

As with most of the recommendations in this book, budgeting your practice expenses for a predictable profit is a good idea in good times. In hard times it becomes a must. While in good times, for example, we would never look to cut costs by reducing an item like bonuses, I could imagine that in really bad times, we might look at lowering or even eliminating bonuses, in order to preserve salaries. My point is that without a budget in place and working for you now, you have little chance of monitoring and controlling costs when you have to. If you don't have an office budget, start one. If you don't know how, get your accountant to help you, but do it!

A word about net profit (or the "bottom line"). There has always been considerable confusion when dentists attempt to compare net profit percentages. I've discovered that the confusion arises through a comparison of one man's apples with another's oranges. If we wish to compare net profits, we need to be comparing the same things, and that requires sorting out expenditures to arrive at the "real" cost of running the practice. For example, pension contributions for your staff are a "real" cost of doing business, but the doctor's pension contribution is not. Taking your staff to lunch is a "real" business expense; some other entertainment costs may not be. The doctor's share of health insurance premiums is truly part of his compensation and should not be included in the "real" cost of operation. When we get down to actual business expenses, we can calculate percentages and compare with one another in a realistic way that makes some sense and is useful.

FEES

In examining the role that fees play in the overall financial structure of your practice, I think it's important to first ask the question, "What do my fees really mean?" I have found that most of my colleagues assume that their patients are aware of not only their fee schedules, but also how their fees relate to other dentists in their area. Some investigative work on my part has revealed to me (even with the small sample in my study) that: (a) aside from the fees for repetitive procedures, like a prophy or an examination, most patients have little idea of what we charge per surface for restorations or what a molar root canal costs; and (b) except for the "shoppers," they have just as little awareness of what our competition charges. They are actually much more interested in what percentage of their bill will be paid for by their insurance carrier.

Furthermore, most of us believe that our fees will have a major influence on the patient's decision-making process–that if our fee is "too high," they will say "no." To illustrate the fallacy in that thinking, I'll tell two stories.

When I first started my practice and went about creating a fee schedule, I consulted with some dentists in my neighborhood and tried to find a middle range for my fees that would not be out of line with any of them. The only fee that was really out of line was my fee for full dentures. I hated doing dentures, and I had the notion that if my denture fee was astronomical, I wouldn't have to make any. So, in the days when amalgam fillings were $5 per surface and a crown was $75, I set my denture fee at $500! Would it surprise you to learn that I did no fewer dentures than any of my competitors? The fee didn't make any difference. That was the beginning of my understanding that my fee has very little to do with patient acceptance of a service. If the patient wants the treatment that you've proposed, he will find a way to pay your fee.

Last year, at a meeting of the Management Study Group, we did a comparison of our fee schedules. Most of us found that we were all within a certain range for each service that we provide, until we came to composite restorations. One of our members had a per surface fee for composites that was twice as much as anyone's in the room and almost triple some members'. When questioned about the discrepancy, his answer was that he found it took him so much longer to do a good composite than anything else he did, and he felt justified in getting that fee. Did he do fewer composites than anyone else in the group? No, he just got paid more for them.

So then, what does your fee represent? It is a statement of a monetary value that you place on a service that you provide. If you believe that your crowns are worth $1,000, you should receive that fee. If you honestly feel that your single root canal is worth $150, that's what you should charge. I would hope that all of your fees are, deservedly, higher than anyone else's in your area, as an expression of the kind of quality service and care you provide for your patients. And if you find or feel that you only deserve a below-average fee for what you do, I hope you'll go out and upgrade what you do and how you do it, in order to justify a healthy fee schedule.

Now let's look at the business of fees in a bad economic environment. Unless you've been practicing for more than 45 or 50 years, you've spent your entire professional life in an inflationary spiral. Yes, there have been occasional recessions, but in actuality, they've been nothing more than temporary slow-downs or halts in the upward curve of wages and prices. In the worst of those recessionary periods, you've probably never decreased your fees or had to lower salaries. So if we do enter into a sustained recession and if it does go on for more than a year or so, we will all be operating in an economic atmosphere with which we have no personal experience.

Under those circumstances, we will, as small business owners, be faced with situations and decisions we've never confronted before. What will you do when the competition reduces fees by 10 percent? How will you react when, even by maintaining the same level of "busyness," your collections drop off? Obviously, we'll have to take a "wait and see" attitude on this issue, but the best preparation in this area is to be very aware of what's going on around you and to have contingency plans ready to put into effect. For example, if revenues decrease by 10 percent and most of it is in increased receivables, I'll do nothing. If the drop is 15 percent or more, I'll eliminate bonuses or drop one staff person. Going through the possibilities will at least mentally prepare you for decisions I hope we never have to make.

At this point, some serious contemplation of your options under various circumstances is about the best you can do. But what should we do right now? There are those who believe that, prior to deflation, we will go through a period of hyper-flation, with prices and wages rapidly shooting up, out of control. In the past, when that has happened, the government has often responded with wage and price controls. If your fees have not kept up with what's happening around you, they could be "frozen" at a level that could work to your disadvantage.

Examine your fee schedule and be certain that you are at least somewhat above average. I also plan to review our fees on a six-month basis, rather than annually, and may eventually reevaluate them on a quarterly basis.

CHAPTER FOUR

VOLUME VS. QUALITY

I've listened for years to the debate among colleagues over "volume" versus "quality" as if the two were mutually exclusive. I don't believe they are. Some of the best dentists I know are also the fastest. Doing something slowly doesn't mean doing it well. If you needed a crown, would you want your dentist to penetrate quickly to the D-E junction and strip away the enamel with a rapid counter-clockwise sweep, or would you prefer that he grind away the enamel, a quarter millimeter at a time, with a rough diamond? The really good clinicians not only set high standards for the quality of the work they do, they also know how to work efficiently and quickly. Many of the top dentists in the country do high quality dentistry, and they do it for a lot of people.

Actually, I find that the really good operators–the ones who are quality oriented and fast–seem to create a strong demand for their services. So, in my mind, there is no debate over quality vs. volume: the two can go very comfortably hand-in-hand.

Here's how I've always looked at the issue: I'm constantly looking for ways to improve the quality of what I do, as well as the efficiency with which I do it. I want to do good dentistry and I want a volume practice, at the same time. I've always thought of volume as "security." In good times, it's what provides me with an above average income.

In hard times, it's the cushion that makes me not as concerned or vulnerable as I might be. Here's what I mean: If hard times come, and all the practices in my area suffer a 20 percent decrease in business (busyness), I can absorb that more easily than a low volume practice. Now, I know there are some low volume/very high fee practices to which that doesn't apply, but for the average general practice, building up the volume in good times can provide some security when the economy turns sour.

By way of example (and this may sound cruel or harsh) the owner of a volume practice with one or more associates, faced with fewer patients and/or production, might choose to reduce the hours of or even let associates go, so as to maintain his own productivity. A practice whose volume is sufficient to authentically keep two hygienists busy might be forced to let one go in hard times, but would then be reduced to a "normal" (one hygienist) level. So I do believe there's security in numbers, and I want to spend some time looking at ways to increase the volume of your practice now in preparation for what may lie ahead.

BUYING AN "OLD" PRACTICE

This next section is worth ten times the cost of this book–if not more– and it's my own idea!

About four years ago, I sat down and wrote the following letter:

> Dear Dr. _____,
>
> I don't know where you see yourself in your professional career, but if you are now or in the near future considering the possibility of retirement, I'd like to meet with you to discuss continuing care for your patients.
>
> I have a proposal to make that could be of interest and benefit to you and to the people whom you've served.
>
> My receptionist, Lynne, will be calling in a few days to see if you are interested in getting together.
>
> Hope to meet with you soon,
> Mort Ehudin

I sent that letter out to every dentist in my area who was 55 years old or older. When Lynne made her follow-up calls, she got no takers, but about a year later I got a call from a colleague who practices in a medical building just down the street. He wanted to meet for lunch.

Since I hadn't had any contact with him in almost fifteen years, I assumed it had something to do with my letter, and I was right. Along with four other dentists in his building, he had been a recipient. He told me at lunch a few days later that one of the "boys" was really insulted by that letter. "What does that guy think I am, an old geezer?" he had remarked. But my lunch partner (let's call him Dr. Davis) wasn't offended at all. Actually, he said, he hadn't given retirement a lot of thought until that letter came, but it prompted him to evaluate his situation. He was down to seeing patients about two and a half days a week. He really didn't need the income anymore and was really just waiting for his wife to get out of the real estate business so they could move down to Florida. My letter was read at their dinner table the night it arrived, and it sparked a discussion about the "when" of their move. It now looked like they had arranged things so that they could go whenever they wanted, and he was ready to hear my proposal.

Here's what I told Dr. Davis:

"If you want to get the most out of the sale of your practice, you should look for some young guy to buy you out and take over the practice."

"Well, I've looked into that," he replied, "and the equipment is so old nobody really wants it, and the location isn't anything anyone would pay to get, so that doesn't seem to be a real possibility."

"Dr. Davis," I responded, "I'm also not interested in your equipment or your location, but I am interested in providing continued care to your patients, and I'm willing to compensate you for the good will you've created with those people. Here's what I'm ready to offer you. You mail out a letter to all of your patients-of-record announcing your retirement and informing them that you have selected me to continue their dental care. We'll put in my phone number and let them know that they should call my office to make their next recall appointment. I'll pay you $100 for every one of your patients who shows up at my office for a recall appointment."

Dr. Davis figured he had about 300 to 500 active patients, and the idea sounded a lot better to him than just closing the door and walking away. He even made the suggestion that, when he closed his office, we have the phone company make his phone ring in my office.

Well, we firmed up the deal in writing, his letter went out, and we became the benefactors of the best thing we ever did for our practice.

Dr. Davis had practiced in our area for 34 years. He was adored by his patients, who were primarily in the 50 to 65 age range and, for the most part, were from the "establishment" of Fort Washington. While they loved Dr. Davis, they all knew that over the last five or ten years he had "slacked off" and really hadn't been taking very good care of them. He had been doing a lot of patch-up work and putting off doing procedures that he didn't feel up to doing anymore.

The patients who came to us from Dr. Davis could be characterized as follows: They were universally nice people. They were extremely loyal to him and willing to transfer that loyalty if justified. They needed a lot of good dentistry, and they knew it! They were all in a position to pay for complete care.

Over the course of the following year, we saw about 100 of Dr. Davis' former patients, and two years later, they continued to dribble in. For the $10,000 we paid Dr. Davis, we got to do more than $75,000 in dental services, but the best part has been that when those people saw what a modern dental practice was like, they became our best missionaries in the community. I really don't know how to calculate the value of that deal to our practice. In terms of production and referrals and bringing so many nice people into our office, it was a bonanza!

I'm negotiating with another "Dr. Davis" at the moment, and I only hope it goes as well.

If you're looking to expand your practice volume quickly, I can't think of a faster or better way than to find an "old" practice to buy. Buying an old practice aside, all other attempts to expand the volume of a practice come under the umbrella called "marketing," so let's examine some options.

CHAPTER FIVE

INTERNAL/EXTERNAL MARKETING

Rick Kushner wrote a wonderful article for Dental Economics last year titled "Hook and Glue." He made the point in his article that many dentists swing back and forth between internal and external marketing schemes, as the current trend goes from one to the other. He goes on to say that a well-rounded marketing plan should contain both, but that external marketing (advertising), without a strong internal marketing plan in place, is a waste. Kushner likes to think of advertising as a "hook" to bring new people into your practice, but you must have a good internal marketing program to "glue" them to the practice and turn them into patients. I couldn't agree with him more.

Over the years, I've tried my share of advertising schemes with mixed results. Nothing that I've tried has been spectacular, and enough of them have been horrible flops to make me think twice about using advertising at all. Placing ads in local newspapers, yearbooks, show programs and on bowling score sheets is a waste. A well-designed and large enough ad in the Yellow Pages, on the other hand, can be very effective. The difference between a successful Yellow Pages ad and one that gets poor results requires professional advice. Before you spend a lot of money on a phone directory, hire someone who knows what he or she is doing (Fig. 5–1).

Mailings to new residents in the area inviting them to become

Four Critical Things to Know Before you Pick a Dentist in Fort Washington:

1. Your new dentist should be **COMPETENT** and **EXPERI-ENCED** in all phases of dentistry, including children's dentistry, denture, crowns and bridges, root canal treatment, gum therapy, as well as artificial tooth implants and cosmetic dentistry.

2. He or she should provide **GENTLE DENTAL CARE**, using all the most up-to-date techniques to make your treatments as easy and comfortable as possible. He or she should also be **COMPASSIONATE** and really **LISTEN** to you.

3. He or she should be oriented toward **PREVENTION** of dental problems, always aware that it is far better (and less costly) to prevent trouble rather than fix it.

4. Your new dentist should be **CONCERNED** about your problems and give **EMERGENCIES** top priority. He or she should be available when you are in need and know that you can't wait when you're in pain.

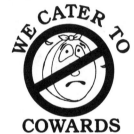

COWARDS

MORTON M. EHUDIN, D.D.S.

In the Livingston Square Mall

248-2020

Serving Oxon Hill/Ft. Washington Since 1965

Fig. 5–1 Yellow Pages Advertisement (quarter-page)

patients have, generally speaking, produced disappointing results. I recently moved to a new home and in the first two months was besieged by "invitations" to partake of a wide variety of services – everything from dentistry (three) to dry cleaning and pet grooming. Quite frankly, I doubt if I would choose any of those services based on a mailer, but perhaps I'm jaded. We have used direct mail to send out offers of examination and full series x-rays for five dollars to the ZIP codes around the office. We can just about count on one-half of one percent response. It's an expensive way to market, and I'm not really sure it's worth the money and the trouble, but we use it to give a boost to the traditionally slow months of the year. The same goes for discount coupons in the packets that are mailed out. It does get some response, but probably not worth the cost. I've just about come to the conclusion that, whereas direct mail marketing was very successful in its early days, at this point people are inundated with "junk mail" and, for the most part, don't even look at it.

Other external marketing attempts that we've used with great expectations and small results are doing "toothbrushing" talks to elementary school children, giving talks about dentistry to local clubs and churches, participating in an area health fair, publicizing "lost children" ID chips (bonded into molars), doing free oral cancer checks in a local mall, participating in Doctors with a Heart, sponsoring a soccer team, and handing out our business cards wherever we go.

Does it sound as if I'm disillusioned by external marketing schemes? Well, yes and no. The truth is that we consistently attract 50 to 60 new patients a month into the practice, and I really don't know exactly where they come from. Oh, we ask them, and some of them tell us, but I've become convinced that it's not all that clear-cut. I think a lot of what's behind a referral is name recognition, and the more places and the more ways your name is "out there" in your community, the better your chances are of getting referrals. So when a new patient says she was "referred" by Betty Smith, that might actually have been the last event in a chain that brought her to your office. Maybe she saw your booth at the Health Fair, and maybe her husband heard you speak at the Rotary Club, and maybe she got a mailer (but didn't use it), and then Betty Smith told her she ought to come see you. So we keep doing external marketing, even though it's often difficult to see direct results; somehow I feel that it gives us name recognition and thereby an edge in winning referrals. And if times get tough, I'll be looking for the most cost-effective ways to keep our name circulating as the place to go for dental care in Fort Washington. But just getting your name around in your neighborhood is not really enough. At the same time, you need to differentiate yourself from all the other practices in your area. And you can't do that by claiming that you are better than anyone else. That's unethical. What I'm really talking about here is what the advertising people call "positioning in the market place." That means identifying and carving out a niche for yourself and then promoting that niche to the public.

What is your practice orientation? What do you do best? What do you want to be "known" for in your community? Are you heavily oriented toward prevention? Are you interested in attracting the people in your geographic area who desire good preventive care? Then all of your external marketing should be directed toward that segment of the population. You should definitely be represented at local health fairs, and you should be giving talks in your area on the benefits of prevention, and you should be giving out floss all over town (with your name on it).

Are you practicing in or near a retirement community? Is your practice geared to take care of the special needs of the elderly? Is that the part of the population that you would love to have flocking to your office? Then that's what you need to promote, and that's how you need to orient your external marketing.

Just promoting your practice as one more "general dentist" or even "family dentist" doesn't give a prospective patient, out looking for a dentist, any particular reason to choose your practice over any other. Your external marketing needs to provide that reason. And it needs to be consistent and repetitive. Marketing people claim that most people don't even become aware of a piece of advertising until they've seen it 27 times. Twenty-seven times! And we send out a mailer and wonder why it didn't do us any good.

In our practice, we decided years ago that what we did best was convert people who were afraid of dentistry into good patients. Our whole practice is oriented around that theme. We use nitrous-oxide analgesia routinely, stereo headphones, and anything else that will make our patients comfortable and at ease. I've spent a lot of time mastering the art of giving painless injections. Our chairside assistants and hygienists are extremely compassionate and caring people who do a lot of hand holding and shoulder squeezing. Everything that they and I do for our patients has been examined in detail, with an eye toward making the procedure as "gentle" as possible. Our reputation is just that – that we don't hurt anyone. And that's where most of our patient referrals come from. People that we have converted from dental "cowards" into "heroes," go out and tell the people they know like themselves to come see us.

We really enjoy making those conversions for the great satisfaction of bringing someone who has stayed away back to dentistry, but also those are the very people who need our services the most. People who have avoided dentistry for years and years, once convinced that they have nothing to fear, are not only extremely appreciative, but they are also ready and willing to go ahead with treatment recommendations. Just prove to them that you won't hurt them and the reaction is most often, "Doc, do whatever you have to get me fixed up." Isn't that the

M. M. EHUDIN, DDS, PA
GENERAL DENTISTRY

9500 LIVINGSTON ROAD   **COWARDS**
LIVINGSTON SQUARE MALL
FORT WASHINGTON, MARYLAND 20744
301-248-2020

COMPLETE FAMILY DENTAL CARE

- CHILDREN AND ADULTS
- DENTURES AND PARTIAL DENTURES
- CROWNS AND BRIDGES
- ROOT CANAL TREATMENTS
- GUM TREATMENTS
- ARTIFICIAL TOOTH IMPLANTS
- COSMETIC VENEERS AND BLEACHING
- FULL PREVENTIVE CARE
- MINOR ORTHODONTICS

Fig. 5–2 Business Card (front and back)

kind of patient we all dream about? But it takes some work to develop that kind of reputation in a community. That's exactly the one we've managed to cultivate, and we know that it gets around by word of mouth.

When we decided to do external marketing, that was the message that we decided to get out into the community. That if you were afraid of the dentist, we were the place for you to go. That we specialize in taking care of people just like you. So every piece of external marketing that goes out of our office carries that same message – perhaps in different ways – but the message is always the same (Fig. 5–2). That is our niche. That's our position in the market place. That's the reason we want to give a prospective patient for choosing us. And it works.

MORTON M. EHUDIN, DDS, PA

9500 LIVINGSTON ROAD
FORT WASHINGTON, MARYLAND 20744
301 248-2020

Our Anniversary Gratitude

Spring 1990

It hardly seems possible, but 1990 marks the 25th anniversary of our dental practice. We've certainly come a long way from that little two-bedroom apartment in Wilson Towers, which many of you can remember. And, while we've grown in size, we've worked hard to preserve the human values that we feel make our practice unique.

We've fixed a lot of teeth over the years, but what really keeps us going are the wonderful personal relationships that we have with you-our patients.

So we want to pause for a moment, on the occasion of our 25th year, to re-dedicate ourselves to providing you with the very highest quality of dental care, and to thank you for your loyalty, your trust in us, and your continued support. Every time you refer a relative or a friend to us, we accept that expression of your confidence with the utmost gratitude.

Warm regards,

Morton M. Ehudin, D.D.S
and Staff

Fig. 5–3 Anniversary Gratitude Letter

Enough about the "hook." Where I think it's really "at" as far as generating large numbers of patient referrals is internal marketing. That sounds so "Madison Avenue." I really like to think of internal marketing as just "taking care of people." It's just the combination of all the things we do to make our patients feel special. (Fig. 5–3). It goes right back to the first law of business that my father gave me on opening

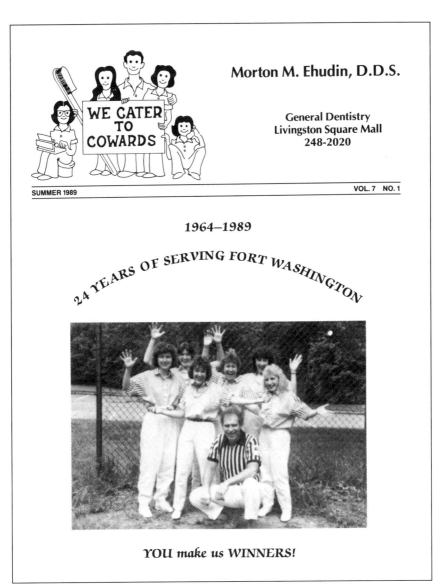

Morton M. Ehudin, D.D.S.

WE CATER
TO
COWARDS

General Dentistry
Livingston Square Mall
248-2020

SUMMER 1989

VOL. 7   NO. 1

1964–1989

24 YEARS OF SERVING FORT WASHINGTON

YOU make us WINNERS!

Fig. 5–4 Newsletter

day: Take good care of people, and they'll take good care of you. (You can have everything you want in life, if you give enough other people what they want.)

Making people feel special is something we work at all the time (Fig. 5–4). When I talk to my staff about making people feel special, I like to talk about my experience of going to see my physician. He's a personal friend and (coupled with the fact that I'm a fellow health professional) I really get special treatment when I go to his office. It starts on the phone, when his receptionist (knowing that I'm a busy doctor) is willing to work me in whenever it's convenient for me. None of this "He only does examinations in the morning" for me. I just about get to name my time. And then when I show up there, I don't have to sign in because they all know me, and I never have to sit out there in the waiting room with the peasants. If he's not ready to see me, I get to wait in his private office. And they always bring me coffee. And they remember that I take cream and no sugar. And I never have to fill out insurance forms; they take that up with my office manager. And I have the doctor's private number at home. In other words, they treat me like I'm somebody special, not like just another patient. When you and I are able to make our patients feel that way, we've got it made. They'll send us more new patients than we know what to do with. In hard times, we're going to need "good friends of the practice" like that, but we need to start cultivating them now.

We want our patients to feel "special," and we want them to feel like they "belong" in our practice. For our young patients we do that with our No Cavities Club. There's not a kid who comes to us who doesn't check out the Polaroid photos on that board to see their own picture and to see who else they know who comes to us. It makes them feel important, and it make them feel like they "belong," For adults, we have Our Book of Smiles, a collection of full face photos of our patients smiling. People just love to look at people smiling, and they love to look for people they know, and having their picture in our book makes them feel they "belong." We've also used our quarterly newsletter to promote that sense of "belonging." The following lead article appeared in a summer issue:

ARE WE THE "CORNER STORE" OF THE 1990s?

As we go into the fifth year of sending out our practice newsletter, something has come to our attention that we find worthy of comment.

For those of us old enough to remember back 30 or 40 years, neighborhoods were different then. First, they were smaller, and most things were within walking distance. Neighborhood stores and shops were small, and people were "known" there. Those establishments were not only places to do business, they were also places to meet friends and neighbors, to catch up on local news, and to develop a sense of "community." In those smaller neighborhoods people had a feeling of "belonging."

By contrast, today's neighborhoods are large, spreadout, and just about nothing is in walking distance. Few of us are "known" at the closest Giant or People's or Safeway. It's no longer easy to have a sense of belonging anywhere. But here's what we've noticed. Our reception area, more and more, seems to be a place where friends and neighbors "bump into each other." It seems to be a place where people in our community are "known" and where there is a feeling of "belonging." Perhaps we should get rid of the modern furniture and put in a wood stove and some cracker barrels! Anyway, if our practice can be something more to the community than just a place to get good dental care, well that makes us feel good.

The purpose of our practice is to provide a safe, warm, friendly environment within which our patients can receive quality dental care at reasonable cost.

Twenty years ago, I attended a lecture on practice building given by Bob Levoy, and he asked the question, "What makes someone refer a friend or a relative to you?" Most of the responses were "if they're satisfied." But Bob said, "No. Being 'satisfied' means getting what you paid for, and people don't get excited enough about 'being satisfied' to go out and make a recommendation. What makes people enthusiastic enough to make a recommendation is if they got something more than they expected, if they got more than they bargained for, if what they received went beyond their expectations, if they got more than what they feel they paid for."

That was a very powerful thought, and it's one that I've consciously used throughout my career. I've always looked for ways to make my patients feel that they got more from our doctor-patient relationship than they expected, and it has never failed to pay off. About four years ago, we held a series of staff meetings to answer the following question: For each type of appointment that a patient might have in our practice, what can we do to go beyond what the patient expected? We looked at the hygiene appointment, and the recall appointment, and the crown and bridge appointment, and the endodontic appointment, and the denture appointment, etc. Here are some of the things we came up with: We've always given our new patients a toothbrush and a floss sample at their first hygiene appointment, but, as a result of our "brainstorming" session, we

COWARDS

Dr. Morton M. Ehudin
Livingston Square Mall
9500 Livingston Road
Fort Washington, Maryland 20744
248-2020

Personal Oral Hygiene Instruction Sheet

PLAQUE - Dental plaque is a thin film of bacteria that adheres strongly to your teeth, especially around your gum line and in between your teeth. Plaque causes dental decay, gingivitis and periodontal (gum) disease. Proper removal is essential to good oral health and can only be effectively accomplished by a physical means, i.e., brushing and flossing.

BRUSHING - Use a soft toothbrush, as a hard brush can damage tooth enamel. The areas to be cleaned with the toothbrush are: (a)the biting surfaces in the pits and grooves; (b)the tongue and cheek sides of the teeth; and (c)the space between the gums and the teeth and place the toothbrush at a 45 degree angle towards the gum line. Applying light pressure, move the brush in a circular motion. Brush after every meal and before bedtime be sure to change to a new toothbrush every two to three months.

FLOSSING - Tear off a piece of floss about two feet long. Wrap each end around the middle fingers of both of your hands, leaving your thumb and index finger free to aid in holding the floss. Keep your fingers as close together as possible, using 1/2 to 1 inch of floss in between your teeth. The closer together you hold your fingers, the easier it is to control the floss. The following illustrations show how to hold the floss in different areas of the mouth.

How to hold the floss   Upper teeth   Lower teeth

Slip the floss between each pair of teeth by drawing it gently back and forth. Once between the teeth, move the floss up and down along the tooth surfaces while at the same time wrapping it around the tooth as much as possible. Carry the floss under the gum until you feel definite resistance without discomfort. Your gums may bleed slightly and become tender during the first two weeks. This soon ceases and the previously inflamed tissue rapidly heals. You should floss your teeth at least once a day.

1. Brush daily after each meal and before bedtime.
2. Use dental floss daily.
3. Have a cleaning and check-up every six months.

Fig. 5–5 Oral Hygiene Instructions

had plastic carryall bags made up (with our logo on the front), and we now include toothpaste samples, disclosing tablets, and a write up on oral hygiene. Our new denture patients get a carryall with a booklet about their prosthesis, a denture bath (with our logo on top), a denture brush and paste and cleansing tablets, and a pocket mirror in a plastic pouch (with our logo on it) so they can see how nice they look. When a frightened

COWARDS

Dr. Morton M. Ehudin
Livingston Square Mall
9500 Livingston Road
Fort Washington, Maryland 20744
248-2020

What Is A Root Canal?

If it were possible to divide one of your front teeth in half and open it up; you would see a narrow space that runs the length of the tooth. That space houses the nerve of the tooth. If the nerve dies or is injured beyond its ability to heal itself, it must be removed or the tooth will form an abscess. The removal of the nerve, and the cleaning, sterilizing and filling of the nerve space is called ROOT CANAL THERAPY. The treatment usually takes two visits and most of the time is no more difficult to have done than a filling.*

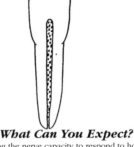

What Can You Expect?

Other than not having the nerve capacity to respond to hot or cold sensations, a root canal tooth is like any other tooth. It can even get a cavity, and needs to be brushed and flossed like any other tooth.

After the first visit, if you had been experiencing tooth aches or severe reaction to hot or cold, the tooth should be either totally free of discomfort or at least much improved. Between the first and second visits, it is a good idea to avoid chewing on the tooth being treated. Some soreness or tenderness to either biting pressure or tapping on the tooth can be expected but if the tooth feels "high" or is very sensitive to biting, it probably needs to have the bite adjusted. If you become aware that the temporary filling in the root canal opening has come out or has been pushed down into the opening, it's important that it be replaced as soon as possible. Call us if you have a problem or any concerns about the treatment.

The fee for root canal therapy is determined by the number of canals in the tooth and is based on a maximum of two visits for completion. Unusual situations that require additional appointments may carry with them an additional fee of $50.00-100.00 The fee for composite, amalgam or crown restorations to restore decay or breakdown of the tooth are unrelated procedures and are additional.

*When Root Canal Therapy (RCT) is complete, the tooth is no longer able to react to hot or cold or to relay pain sensations. Root canal teeth, however, are drier than normal teeth and because they are more brittle, usually need to be covered by a crown to prevent breakage. The decision to crown a root canal tooth is made on a tooth-by-tooth basis.

Fig. 5–6 What is a Root Canal?

patient gets through a first treatment appointment and lets us know how easy it was, we give him a coffee mug with our logo on it. It's kind of cute, and it always gets a smile and a "thank you." Surgical and endodontic patients receive a baggie with pain medication and gauze and printed instructions explaining exactly what was done and why, and what they need to do or be aware of (Figs. 5–5, 5–6, and 5–7). Those are not "stock"

COWARDS

Dr. Morton M. Ehudin
Livingston Square Mall
9500 Livingston Road
Fort Washington, Maryland 20744
248-2020

Owner's Manual for Crowns and Bridgework

Whether you've just received an individual crown(cap) or crowned teeth supporting replacement teeth, we feel that it's important for you to know about your treatment and what you need to do to protect the investment you've made in your mouth.

What Was Done and Why?

If you could take a tooth apart, you would find it has two parts-an inner core of dentin and a hard outer layer of enamel. When a tooth is trimmed for a crown, we essentially remove the outer enamel layer-or its equivalent in filling. After trimming, the remaining stump looks like a miniature of the original tooth.

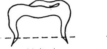

original tooth   trimmed tooth

The finished crown consists of a gold alloy thimble, which very accurately fits the stump and acts to support and hold the remaining tooth together. Porcelain is baked over the metal thimble to simulate tooth enamel.

When crowns are used as supports to replace missing teeth, the replacement tooth(or teeth) is welded to the support crowns. This combination of supporting crowns and replacement teeth is called a fixed (or permanent) bridge.

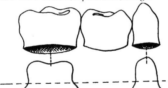

All crowns are attached to the tooth stump by an epoxy-like cement, with the borders of the crown tucked up under the gum. When crowns or bridges have been accurately adjusted, they should feel comfortable and in harmony with your bite. You should notice no bumping into or tripping over your crown, no matter how you move your jaw around. If you are aware of anything unusual about the bite of your crown, please let us know right away. Other than possibly the shape or form of your crown, you should not have to "get used to it."

Your crowns need the same kind of care as the rest of your teeth. They need to be brushed and flossed daily. Since floss cannot be passed between crowns and replacement teeth on a bridge, we'll show you how to use a floss threader to get under the replacement tooth.

Fig. 5–7 Owner's Manual for Crowns and Bridges

instructions. I wrote them, and they're printed on our stationary, with our logo. And every baggie that we give out also has a few of our business cards in it.

We have a TV in the reception area, because a survey of our patients told us that's what they wanted. We put a phone in the reception room, also, for patients to use. It isn't used very often, and no one has taken advantage of it, but we know the thought is appreciated. Every one of our patients is given a carnation at the end of every appointment. At special times of the year, we substitute something else for the flowers, like a tree ornament at Christmas time, or an apple in the fall, or a painted Easter egg, or shamrock appliques for St. Patrick's Day.

Those are the things we do to make our patients feel special at every appointment, but you and your staff should sit down in a series of meetings and figure out what you want to do to make every patient at every appointment feel like they got more than they paid for.

Can you imagine how our new patients feel when they walk out of our office having had their blood pressure taken, an oral cancer check, thorough oral hygiene instructions, careful scaling and polishing, with their baggie full of hygiene "goodies" in one hand and a carnation in the other? And they thought they were just coming for a cleaning! It doesn't happen every time, but do you think it's possible that that patient just might tell her neighbor, or the people in her car pool, or her sister about the wonderful new dentist she found? And if she's not the kind of person who usually thinks of making referrals for anything, we give her the idea by sending out a note.

I hand write a similar note (that's right, I do them by hand) to every new patient (Fig. 5–8). The one line that's always the same is the last one. It's our promise, and at the same time, it's a direct request for referrals. Lots of people – even people who are excited about your practice – would just never think of telling anyone about you. That last line can give them the idea. I've always maintained that internal marketing was a "game of inches." There aren't many big winners. It's a little gain here and a little there, and all together it's a program that produces results. But if there is one thing that we do that gives us traceable referrals, it's that welcome letter to new patients. I used to think that my referrals came from people that I had done a lot of dentistry for, and who were pleased with my work. It took me a long time to figure out that people make referrals when they're excited and enthusiastic and "hot," and that happens right in the beginning of their relationship with your practice. After a time, the most enthusiastic missionaries lose their fervor. Our welcome letter asks for referrals when a new patient is "hot."

Asking our patients for referrals is definitely the most successful single thing we do in generating a high number of new patients. If there is a "second best," it's getting referrals from other professionals. Cultivating the friendship of a pharmacist or physician in your area can bring you a steady stream of "quality" referrals. By "quality" I don't

MORTON M. EHUDIN, DDS, PA
9500 LIVINGTON ROAD
FORT WASHINGTON, MARYLAND 20744
301 248-2020

COWARDS

Janet —

Just a note to welcome you to
our practice, and to thank you for
choosing me as your dentist. My aim
is to get you fixed up as quickly and
easily as possible — and then see that
you stay that way!

My staff and I are planning to
take such good care of you that you'll
tell everybody you know to come see us.

See you soon —

Dr. Ehudin

Fig. 5–8 Handwritten Welcome Letter

mean superior in any way, since I'm absolutely convinced that there's
no such thing as the "wrong kind of patient." By "quality" I do mean
a patient who comes to you from a referral source that has established
your reputation up front. When my physician sends me a new patient
(and he sends me a lot!), I don't need to establish my reputation with
that person. Dr. Mac has already told him that he's sending him to "the

best," and since he has the reputation of being the best M.D. in Fort Washington, that recommendation carries tremendous weight. So when a "quality" new patient comes to me, my job is really easy. I just need to determine what he needs and tell him. He's already set up to accept my suggestions.

About a year ago, Dr. Mac hired a young man as his physician's assistant. For all the routine things he has to deal with, Donald has now taken over. Since everyone on my staff is a patient at Dr. Mac's practice, we all see Donald for our minor bumps and bruises, colds, flu shots, and hepatitis shots. So we've all gotten to know Donald, and he knows us. The first thing we noticed about Donald was that he was a very nice guy. The second thing we noticed was that he had two of the ugliest gold and plastic crowns on his central incisors that we had ever seen, and his cuspids were longer and pointier than anything you could see on a late Saturday night horror show.

We talked about Donald in a staff meeting and decided he would be a good friend to cultivate, so I sent him a letter and told him that we really appreciated the special attention that he always gave to me and my staff, and that I wanted to thank him by remaking his crowns for him. He was, of course, surprised and delighted, especially with the results, which were quite dramatic – two beautiful porcelain crowns and nicely rounded off cuspids that made him look so much friendlier. When I was finished, Donald said, "Dr. Ehudin, I really appreciate what you've done for me. I just don't know how to thank you." To which I replied, "Donald, it's been my pleasure, and there is something you could do for us. We just love the kind of patients that you and Dr. Mac send to us. They're super nice people, and you always send them with such high recommendations that make it real easy for us to work with them. I know that a lot of your patients rarely even see Dr. Mac since you've been there, so you could do us a big favor by just letting those people know about us when it's appropriate." I know he got the message, and we're already reaping the rewards of our generosity toward him.

If you don't have those kinds of working relationships with good professionals in your area, it's worth spending the time to develop them, and a good way to begin is to establish contact with the physicians of your new patients. We find out, as part of our medical history, which physician our new patient goes to, and then we send him or her a note letting the doctor know that Mrs. Lester has come to us for her dental care and we would appreciate him letting us know if there is anything about her medical background that we should be aware of (Fig. 5–9). Any physician worth his salt will at least be impressed by your thoroughness, and if he's gotten six or seven of your notes over the course of a few months, the door should be open for a "get acquainted" lunch. Since most dentists never bother to ask physicians for referrals, you've got a good chance of getting him to refer to you when you pop the question. Getting him to include a question about the condition of teeth and gums on his medical history is a great way to lead into a possible referral. If a patient indicates that he has dental problems and that he doesn't have a dentist, it's very natural for the physician to make a referral, if you've got him on your side.

Not too long ago, an ambulatory emergency medical facility opened in our neighborhood. We let them know that we respond to emergency calls on a 24-hour basis, and left some of our cards. We also stop by, from time to time, to remind them that we still exist. They get a lot of accident cases, and I just know that, sooner or later, that's going to be a good referral source for us.

Pharmacists are very often the "poor man's doctor." People come to them all the time for medical advice. They're really not supposed to tell people what to do or take, but they do, and they get plenty of dental questions. We've gotten to be very friendly with our pharmacist (mainly by asking his advice on drug selection), and now he adds to his dental advice: "But you should really go see Dr. Ehudin down at the other end of the mall."

Now, I know a lot of dentists who claim they don't want those "emergency toothaches." They think of emergencies as interruptions in their schedule. What they're really saying is that they believe there's a "right kind of patient" and a "wrong kind of patient," and emergency toothaches are the "wrong" kind. In our practice, we've come to see that there's just no way to determine who will be the "right" or "wrong" kind of patient. We love to see emergency patients, and if your practice is going to make it through tough times, you'd better come to love them too. When we get a call from a person in pain, we ask only one question: "How fast can you get here?" In spite of a busy schedule (and we have one just about every day), we're never too busy to get someone out of pain. Even if it means an injection and a seat in the reception area until we can find some time to solve the problem, we stop the hurting. That kind of compassion is what I would want for myself, it's what we give everyone who turns to us for help, and it has brought us a full share of referrals from grateful sufferers. Even the "wrong" kind of patient can be a great source of referral. We've all known the patient who only comes in to have problems taken care of-

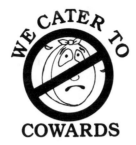

WE CATER TO

COWARDS

Dr. Morton M. Ehudin
Livingston Square Mall
9500 Livingston Road
Fort Washington, Maryland 20744
248-2020

Dear

We are beginning dental treatment on _____,

and would appreciate any information regarding

medical history you think we might need.

Thank you,

Fig. 5–9 Letter to Patient's Physician

not what we would call the "right" kind of patient. But how often have those "wrong" kind referred lots of the "right" kind to us?

Mrs. Bigley has, officially, been a patient of mine for over ten years; but she is certainly not what we would call the "right kind of patient." She only comes in when she has a problem. She has never had a complete examination or a full series of radiographs. She has never even had a prophylaxis. Mrs. Bigley shows up (very often unannounced) when she is in trouble. If the problem can't be fixed easily and inexpensively, she wants to go to the oral surgeon for another extraction. She is definitely the kind of person that no ethically practicing dentist likes to have as a patient, and it would have been with full justification that I could have dismissed her, years ago. And believe me, I have been tempted. I have patched teeth that should have had full coverage, and I have extracted teeth that were periodontally beyond hope. Fortunately, I see Mrs. Bigley about once every two or three years, and that suits me just fine.

About six months ago Mrs. Bigley showed up, on an emergency basis, with an upper lateral incisor that was waving in the breezes. She knew that it had to come out, and for the first time in our over ten-year relationship, she was ready to consider some kind of replacement. This time I insisted on a full set of x-rays, and proposed that I make her an all-acrylic partial denture with wrought wire clasps to replace the soon-to-be-history lateral as well as the missing posterior teeth in that arch.

Mrs. Bigley wanted to know how much the wire clasps would cost compared to no wire clasps. I usually don't find myself getting down to that kind of hair splitting, but I gave her a fee to include clasps and one that did not. As insignificant as the difference was, she opted for "no clasps"; and so, I made her a "flipper" and sent her happily on her way-until the next "emergency."

As usual, this most recent encounter with Mrs. Bigley left me with feelings of frustration and disappointment in not being able to do for a patient what I knew would be my best. On the other hand, I have always believed that I owe it to the community that I serve to provide the best treatment that I can for each patient, within the framework of his or her understanding and acceptance, at the time. To my credit, I have a pretty good track record for converting the Mrs. Bigley's of Fort Washington into understand and accepting patients. And I also know that we can't win them all!

About four months after Mrs. Bigley went home with her new flipper, I was interviewing a new patient, a Mrs. Howard, when I noticed on her information sheet that she was referred to me by (of all people) Mrs. Bigley! I asked how she knew Mrs. Bigley. She said they were neighbors and that she just loved the teeth that I made for her.

I inquired, "What was it that you liked so much?" "Oh," she exclaimed, "They look so natural. Not like false teeth at all. They don't have any of those ugly hooks. I just hate to see those awful hooks on people's teeth. And Mr. Bigley's teeth look just as nice."

Now I never, ever met Mr. Bigley. I didn't even know the man existed, but I accepted the compliment and the information provided, and went on with the interview.

Last week we completed Mrs. Howard's case. We did sixteen units of crown and bridge for her and two precision attachment partial dentures. She was delighted! She had all of her teeth back and no ugly hooks. Just like Mrs. Bigley!

This week Mr. Howard came to see me. He told me his wife wants him to finally get rid of that partial denture with the ugly hooks.

The pay off was a long time in coming (and perhaps it would never have come), but suddenly, all those years of putting up with Mrs. Bigley's emergencies paid off for me. My belief was strengthened that serving the whole community, not just the dentally educated, ultimately builds a stronger practice.

If you don't have your emergency techniques down pat, you should develop your ability to make a quick (but accurate) diagnosis and have at your disposal methods for the quick and efficient relief of pain. Primarily, I believe it's what you owe the public you serve, but if hard times come, you'll need to be known as the place to go for emergency care. And you can't develop that overnight.

Well, I hope I've made my point about building a large volume of patients, but it's not about just getting them in the door. The secret is to rapidly develop every new patient into a source of referral, and then to "bond" each new patient to your practice. By creating a large mass of loyal patients, you give your practice the best possible chance to survive and thrive in any economic climate. That's worth repeating:

By creating a large mass of loyal patients, you give your practice the best possible chance to survive and thrive in any economic climate.

CHAPTER SIX

THE DENTAL TEAM

Not long after I started the practice, in 1966, I hired my first employee, an older (forty-ish) lady who lived in the area and knew just about everybody. She was my assistant/receptionist, and then I took on a part-time hygienist to do the cleanings. There was a little restaurant near the office, where most of the local dentists met for lunch. I used to go there from time to time, but I soon learned to do more listening than talking. I was already doing better than most of them and felt uncomfortable letting them know that. But they were older and more experienced than I was, and I figured I could learn from their experience. I very specifically recall the advice I was given when the "Ranch House Gang" found out that I had two "girls." First, don't ever let them know the facts (income) of the practice. It's none of their business, and it'll just make them jealous. And second, don't get too friendly with them. They'll use it to take advantage of you. That actually sounded like very reasonable advice to me, and I suppose it was the prevalent attitude in 1966.

I suppose I even used that advice for a time, but it didn't take me long to realize that, as the practice grew larger and busier, I couldn't cover all the bases by myself. If I didn't have the kind of rapport with my employees that made them take a personal interest in the success of the practice, it wasn't going to go very far. So I loosened up some and actually got almost friendly with the "girls." But I still kept the secrets of the practice very close to my vest. I even personally wrote out every check that went out of the office.

In 1980, I can't really say that I was looking for something to do with the practice, but I happened to meet a man who consulted with businessmen to teach them how to better lead their companies. Now, I thought I was a pretty good leader already, and I'm sure that the people who worked for me thought that I was a good enough boss to work for, but I decided to hire this guy anyway. He had never worked in a dental practice before, but I soon found out that didn't make a bit of difference. He and I spent five three-hour sessions together going over the principles and techniques of leadership, and then we had another four sessions with me and the staff together. We literally took our boss/employee relationship apart and then put it back together again. And when he was finished, we had gone from what I call "Snow White and the Seven Dwarfs" (where I was Dr. White and they were the dwarfs) to a real dental team.

Not long thereafter, I started reading Avrom King's Nexus newsletter, and when I read his description of "participatory management," I said, "That's it! That's what we've got!" There were five of us then, and we were all equal partners in running the practice. Our staff meetings were actually the meetings of the management committee of the practice. We were "together" as we had never been before. We went on to do the Quest program together and then to become the model practice for the Partners on Purpose program. As a group and as individuals we've given talks and led discussion groups all over our area. My employees are truly my partners in the practice. Knowing that they have a say in the decision making process and that they share in the profits of the practice gives them a vital interest in seeing that we succeed. With eight of us watching over all the details that go into running the practice, the chances for success are just that much greater.

Today, if I were asked to identify the single most significant difference between the successful practices of the 1960s and those of the seventies and eighties, I would say, "the team concept." Whereas the top practices of the fifties and sixties managed to achieve success with the dentist as the superstar and the staff in a very subservient role, in order to achieve success in today's environment, it has become clearly apparent that the dentist cannot do it alone. I can think of no successful contemporary practice in which the doctor does not share not only the management decisions and responsibility, but also the profits of the practice with his staff.

Just as dental school graduates of the sixties and beyond came to understand that a knowledge of business skills had become crucial to success in private practice, today's practitioners have or are coming to understand that personnel management and leadership skills are vital to success in the nineties and beyond. Knowing that, what steps can a dentist take to create the team concept needed to manage the modern practice?

First, I believe he or she needs to examine the various roles the dentist plays within his practice, to sort them out (isolate them) and then learn to use each for maximum efficiency. Here's what I mean: Most dentists, in the context of their practices, wear four different hats. They are the owner, the president of the company, the manager, and the chief technician. It's really important to understand that a dental practice is a rare bird, in that it's unusual to find a business in which one person fills all four positions. In most businesses, for example, the owners (stockholders) never even show up on the premises. They interact with the business by electing a board of directors, who in turn elect a president of the board, who in turn hires a manager, who then hires technicians or workers. In a well-run business each of those functionaries carries out specific duties. In the typical dental practice, the dentist attempts to fulfill them all, simultaneously, and to do it with his nose buried in a small, dark, wet hole.

Am I suggesting that we dentists give up some or all of those roles? No. Each one is vital to the success of the practice, but I've found it extremely helpful to understand what the functions of each role are and to consciously perform in each role separately. What I mean by that, for example, is that when I'm performing an ownership role – like meeting with the company's lawyer – I should not be mentally reviewing my crown preparation procedures. Now that sounds like a ridiculous example, doesn't it? And yet, for the dentist who has not learned to separate his various roles, what do you think he's thinking about when he's deeply involved in a crown preparation? See if this sounds familiar to you:

(Remember now that our dentist in this example is in his chief technician mode, running his handpiece at 250,000 or 300,000 RPM and making the vital preparation decisions that will ultimately affect the fit and contour and occlusion of the restoration he's committed to provide.)

Let's get inside his head and see what's going on.

"Got to take some more off that lingual occlusal plane. I wonder if my next patient is here yet. If she isn't, maybe I should stop for a minute and check the hygiene patient.   There, that looks like enough clearance. Darn, today's the eighth of the month, and I don't think Janice got the bills out from last month yet. I better talk to her about that. And I don't think she sent off the rent check either. Wish that tongue would stay out of the way! Did Peggy call in that order for alginate? Gotta ask her about that at lunch time. At the rate this morning's going, I doubt if we'll get a lunch. I wonder how Mrs. Crampton is doing after her root canal yesterday. Somebody should call her. That should do it for the lingual margin. I wonder if the Jackson case came back from the lab this morning. I think she's coming in this afternoon, etc., etc."

Considering that that is the kind of conversation that goes on inside our heads at the same time that we are performing excruciatingly complex and precise procedures, it is truly a wonder that so many of us perform as well as we do.

So many of my colleagues tell me how exhausted they are at the end of a day of dentistry, and I know that it's not physical exhaustion – it's mental. After all, we're not digging ditches all day. Our work is not exactly hard physical labor, but I'm convinced that our "end of the day burnout" is a result of trying to do the dentistry and manage everything else at the same time!

Just imagine how much better we could be if we could bring our full concentration to bear on the task at hand! And how much less stressful our days would be! So often I hear my colleagues say, "If I could just be left alone to do the dentistry, without being hassled by all the administrative stuff I have to handle, it would be a snap."

Believe it or not, that's how my days are. When I'm functioning as the manager of the practice, I manage, and when I'm in the role of chief technician, I do dentistry. And the secret is the isolation of my various roles and performing them at specific times.

So, in the morning before I start doing dentistry, and at the end of the day, and perhaps at lunchtime, and most certainly during staff meetings, I manage the practice. But, when I step out of my private office onto what I like to think of as "the stage" of the practice, I take off my manager's hat and put on my technician's hat. With that hat on, I'm 100 percent dentist.

And here's the difference that makes that possible: We're a team.

The only way that I can fully concentrate on dentistry when I'm "on stage" is with the assurance and peace of mind that the staff is managing things. That means that I've given them the responsibility and the authority to manage the practice while I'm doing dentistry. The key there is the authority. Most dentists I know are more than willing to give their staff's responsibility. As a matter of fact, the biggest complaint most of them have is that they won't take any responsibility. But responsibility without authority to act is a powerless and frustrating position to be in, and few employers are willing to give up their authority.

In our practice it works like this: When the practice does well, everyone shares in the rewards. My job in the practice is to do the dentistry (chief technician) and see to it that the practice runs smoothly (manager). As manager I just need to keep monitoring the end product. Are we getting the job done? Are we doing quality dentistry? Are we taking great care of our patients? Are we continuing to get better? Are we in harmony with one another? Are we having a good time? Are we being profitable? But I don't have to be involved with all the details in each of those areas.

I have, in effect, said to my staff, "Since I am your main source of production, I make myself available to you. You can use me as you see fit (within the parameters of the areas that I monitor) to be maximally productive. If you schedule me so that I get to drink lots of coffee and do lots of crossword puzzles, you cheat yourselves. If we run out of alginate and I can't take the impression I need, you lose out on the production. If you didn't follow up on the lab to see that our case was delivered on time, and we have to reschedule a patient, you've wasted my time and hurt your production. If you aren't stimulating referrals from our patients, and we run out of big cases to do, you'll feel it in your paycheck, too."

That's hard for most dentists to do, but this is even harder. When I'm in my "dentist mode," I allow myself to be managed. I give up the right to call the shots and make the decisions about how the day will flow. I've given over that function to my number one assistant, who we call our Treatment Coordinator. Karen is responsible for seeing to it that we stay on schedule, fitting in the five emergencies that we see on an average day, getting us a full hour for lunch and out on time at the end of the day, and pacing me so that I don't tire out.

All the annoying decisions that drive most practitioners up the wall–like which room to go to next, and when to seat the next patient, and where to fit in the emergency, and when to check the hygiene patients–belong to the Treatment Coordinator. As far as my flow in the practice, I just do what she tells me to do, and if we get out late, it's not my fault. "I" don't run over. Sometimes "we" run over. "I" never stick in an emergency just before lunch. Sometimes "we" see an emergency at that time of day.

When I'm in my "dentist mode," I don't get involved with practice management issues. Our Office Manager has the responsibility and the authority to interact with our accountant, lawyer, supply salesman, and banker. If she has a question or a problem, we discuss it during "management time."

So when I'm doing dentistry, I'm doing dentistry, and the only way I know to be able to have that freedom is to allow the staff to essentially run the practice–under my supervision and monitoring.

In giving them that kind of responsibility, I've also had to give them the necessary authority to make decisions (and to make mistakes). In our staff meetings, everyone has one vote, including me. Now, everyone knows that I hold the ultimate veto, but in nine years I've never used it. I did, however, come close at one point.

About six years ago, I was having lunch with the owner of the store right next to our practice in the shopping center. She was complaining that she actually had too much space, and her rent was out of line with the amount of business she was doing. That night, I got the brilliant idea that we could break through the wall between our two areas and take over about 500 square feet from her. It would solve her problem, and we could expand our operation. I even drew up some rough plans, and couldn't wait for our next staff meeting to discuss the project with my partners. You can imagine my reaction when my enthusiastically presented plan went over like a lead balloon. I put the issue to a vote, and I lost, six to two!

For several days I sulked and seriously considered using my veto. After all, it was my practice. If I wanted to expand, I didn't really need their permission. I was probably going to be around here a lot longer than any of them, anyway. But, rather than use the veto, I decided to convince them that they were wrong and should change their votes. So, at the next meeting, I brought up the topic for "further discussion." I had had a whole week to plan my strategy, and I gave a wonderful presentation. When I was finished, one of the chairside assistants, a young lady not known for her oratorical talents, said, "I just don't understand why we need more space. We're really not using the space we already have to the best advantage. If we would just run a wall from here to here, move the lab into that space, and build a supply closet over there, we could have one operatory where the lab is." Just like that. And she was right. That's exactly what we did, saving us the additional rent every month, as well as the costs of construction. With the clarity of hindsight, six years later, I can see it was definitely the right decision. And I can assure you, had it been up to me, we would have made the move next door. Our staff meetings are truly the meetings of the Management Committee of the Practice.

Since we're on the topic, I think it worthwhile to give you the format that we use to conduct our staff meetings. Before we started doing them this way, I found them to be basically a waste of time. We had them irregularly (usually when someone said, "Gee, it's been a long time since we've had a staff meeting." And I would respond, "Yeah, let's schedule one in a couple of weeks.") When we did have one, it was more often than not a "gripe session"–them against me. I always felt under attack and out of control. They apparently had a chance to vent their grievances with "management," but since nothing ever really got resolved, they usually wound up feeling frustrated and hopeless.

In 1980, we made a commitment to have a one-hour staff meeting every week, and I can tell you that that time has become holy to us. Just about nothing, short of an act of God, has stopped us from having our Wednesday meeting. If we have a problem now with staff meetings, it's that they are too short. We never seem to have enough time, so about three or four times a year, we schedule a two-hour session that usually gets used for goal setting or to deal with some major change in our operation. And once a year we schedule an all-day staff meeting to plan out the coming year.

As I said earlier, in our staff meeting everyone has one vote. That makes the process democratic, and to further our aim of participatory management, we rotate the leadership of the meetings: everyone gets a turn to run the meetings. In the meetings, there is no "boss" and there are no "employees," just a gathering of equals.

Here's how we run our meetings:

Each of us has a notebook that we bring to every meeting, and once the chairperson has called the meeting to order, we each write in our books what we've come to call "The Condition of the Practice." That's a short sentence or series of phrases that expresses how we feel the practice is doing, as a whole. Some examples:

"Real busy, but could be more productive. Feel some tension between the front desk and the back. Excited about going to the course next week."

"Things are humming along. Everyone cooperating to make it work. Would like to see more new patients."

"Struggling to keep up with the work load. Feel like we could be getting more support from Hygiene, when they have open time. The overall mood is down from what it should be."

Then we each give the practice a numerical evaluation for the previous week. We write down a number from one to ten (one being "awful" and ten being "wonderful").

At that point in the meeting, we go around the room and each person reads his or her "Condition" and gives his or her number.

This opening exercise gives us an indication of how we're doing as a group, and it also spotlights problem areas. If, for example, three or four people felt that we weren't cooperating with one another or that we weren't taking good care of our patients, we would most certainly spend some time discussing those situations before moving on in the meeting.

In the second part of our staff meeting we focus on the way we're interacting with one another. We do a communication exercise that's designed to clear the air of all the petty resentments that can build up between people in the course of a work week. The exercise is difficult to do, and no one likes doing it, but we all recognize that by doing it we eliminate the possibility of major blowups. We've been doing this exercise religiously for almost ten years now, and I can tell you that it really works. During those ten years, there have been times when we've grown cocky and thought that we were so good that we didn't need to do it anymore. It usually takes about four weeks of not doing the exercise for enough "stuff" to build up in our "team space" that it affects how we work with one another. We had someone teach us to do the communication exercise and "walk" us through it until we could do it alone. I can't do that for you, but I think you can learn it for yourself by following my description. By the way, this exercise works anywhere that people interact with one another. It's a great thing to do around the dinner table once a week.

This is how it's done:

Each member of the group writes down one positive and one negative statement about some other member of the group. The positive and negative statements need not be addressed to the same person. The two statements must follow the format (as given in the examples). Going around the circle, each member first reads his or her negative statement. During the reading of a statement, it's the job of the person being addressed to make absolutely no response. (Rolling eyes, shaking the head, pursing the lips are all responses.) The addressee's job is to simply receive the message. After everyone has read his or her negative statement, the round is made again for the reading of positive statements. (The positives are a lot easier to do than the negatives!)

Here is an example of a negative and a positive statement:

Susan, on Monday morning, when you showed up fifteen minutes late because you stopped to pick up your dry cleaning, I felt abandoned, angry, used, and unsupported.

Ann, on Thursday afternoon, when you finished your patient early and came up front to confirm patients, I felt supported, cared for, appreciated and happy.

We've learned to get over taking a statement directed at us too personally. (It's impossible to not take them somewhat personally!) But after getting over the difficulty of doing the exercise, it becomes possible to start really listening to each other. What begins to evolve for each member of the group is a composite statement of how he needs to be supported by his co-workers. We discovered, for example, that our office manager needs to be supported by not interrupting her without asking for permission and that one of our assistants just needs to know that people are willing to help her out if she gets in a bind, so we support her by asking if she needs help (she usually says "no," but the purpose has been served).

Some of our "negatives" probably would sound like nitpicking if you sat in on one of our staff meetings. (Sally, on Wednesday at lunch time, when you asked Jane if she wanted anything from the deli and you didn't ask me, I felt —) But it's exactly that kind of little stuff that slowly builds up in the relationships between people until one more insignificant event takes place, and an explosion occurs. It's rarely that last event that sets someone off. That last event is the final straw that creates the critical mass needed to go over the edge. If the little stuff gets cleaned out once a week, it never has a chance to build up.

The communication exercise is probably the most important part of our staff meeting. (Fig. 6–1)

We then handle any "Old Business" that needs our attention. We might discuss an issue that we didn't have a chance to finish at the last meeting, or the Office Manager (who acts as our secretary) might ask for the progress report on a certain project, or ask someone if she has carried out an assignment she had accepted.

During "New Business" we discuss topics not dealt with previously.

Our meetings always end with "Good and Welfare." We go around the room, and everyone gets a chance to say, briefly, whatever is on his or her mind that would be to the "good" and "welfare" of the practice. Comments run the gamut from "Thanks, everyone, for helping me out on Tuesday when I wasn't feeling so good" to "Happy to have Susan back from vacation – we missed you" to "I'm having

COMMUNICATION EXERCISE

Positive		Negative	
accepted	interested	anxious	hateful
appreciated	inspired	abandoned	hopeless
admired	invigorated	angry	insulted
affirmed	loved	annoyed	imitated
amused	liberated	bored	ignored
cared for	mellow	criticized	judged
cheered	optimistic	cheated	low
confident	relaxed	concerned	let-down
comfortable	respected	controlled	offended
calm	relieved	confused	put-down
cheerful	reassured	cut-off	perplexed
delighted	recognized	misunderstood	pressured
encouraged	supported	manipulated	rejected
ecstatic	strong	disgusted	repulsed
elated	stimulated	dominated	tense
excited	safe	deceived	teased
fulfilled	thrilled	furious	uptight
grateful	understood	humiliated	used
happy	valued	hurt	unheard
hopeful	worthy	harrassed	

"Yesterday, just before lunch, in the lab, when you _____
I felt _____"

TIME   PLACE   INCIDENT   ACTION   FEELING

Fig. 6–1 Communication Exercise

some problems with my daughter right now and trying not to let it affect my mood here at the office. If anybody thinks I'm not succeeding, please let me know."

There's very often a lot of humor at our meetings, and if we can hold it to a reasonable level, we can go through our format in about one hour. From time to time, something comes up in a meeting that we realize needs more thorough discussion, and occasionally, we've decided ahead of time to devote the entire next staff meeting to that purpose. The important thing is to have regularly scheduled staff meetings and to follow a format that makes them productive.

I'll list our format again, for easy reference.

    I. Condition of the Practice and Numerical Evaluation

    II. Communication Exercise

    III. Old Business

    IV. New Business

    V. Good and Welfare

PURPOSE

While regular and well-run staff meetings are essential ot creating and maintaining a sense of "team" among the dental staff, every team needs a game to play. A clearly defined statement of the "purpose" or the "mission" of the practice lets the players know what game it is they are playing and assists the team in holding their focus on what it is they are up to.

We spent two staff meetings, about seven years ago, writing our statement of purpose. We discussed the meaning of every word in it and looked them up in the dictionary to be sure we were saying what we wanted to say. It was a group effort and wasn't ratified until we were in 100 percent agreement that it was just right for us. We have it framed in our reception room, and it appears on the front page of every one of our practice newsletters. It's our statement to our patients as to what they can expect of us, and our statement to ourselves that we can use as a "touchstone" – a place to come back to when we're not sure where we are or where we're going. We like to read it out loud two or three times a year in a staff meeting, and we often refer to it in making practice-related decisions (to see if a particular action or plan or activity falls within our stated purpose). If you don't have a written statement of the purpose of your practice, I strongly urge you to develop one. Here's ours:

THE PURPOSE OF OUR PRACTICE IS TO CREATE A WARM, SAFE, COMFORTABLE ENVIRONMENT WITHIN WHICH OUR PATIENTS CAN RECEIVE QUALITY DENTAL CARE AT REASONABLE COST, AND OUR EMPLOYEES CAN BE NURTURED, REWARDED, AND CONTINUE TO GROW.

You'll notice that the first part of our statement of purpose is our promise to our patients. The second half is the practice's promise to its employees.

Employees will be "nurtured," "rewarded," and be encourged to "continue to grow." "Nurtured" means taken care of, maintained, trained, educated; and we do that by giving staff members the assurance that their position is secure, that they are worthy members of a health care team, and that they are valuable enough to invest in their continued education. Their continued growth comes through the encouragement to go beyond their job description – to take on more responsibility and to grow as a person. It is of real personal satisfaction to me that I can look at the people who work with me and recognize that, as a result of their being in the practice, they have grown and expanded as human beings. Some of them came to the practice as teenagers and have developed, over the years, into mature, responsible, motivated, self-disciplined young women. All of them have learned and grown in their interpersonal skills. That they are all better people for having worked in the practice is evidence that the practice is fulfilling its purpose.

But the statement of purpose also promises that employees will be "rewarded." I have always considered a salary to be payment for a job performed, but how do you compensate for service above and beyond?

THE BONUS SYSTEM

Some employers use a bonus as an incentive to motivate. I really don't think it works that way. Yes, you can get some people to work harder for more money, but eventually that wears thin. I have always thought of a bonus as a "retroactive" compensation for a job done above and beyond the expected, and there are a thousand ways to give bonuses: everything from "slipping a deserving employee some extra cash" to a formal "profit-sharing" arrangement. Every dentist that I associate with has some kind of a bonus system, and they are all different. We sometimes get into long discussions as to which one works best, and the truth is they all work. But it's not the system that matters, it's the spirit with which a bonus is given. If a bonus is given grudgingly or dutifully or with resentment, it's better not to give one at all.

I look at it this way: I pay an average wage for an average job. My practice is not "average," and I can't have average people working for me, so I only hire people who can perform above average work, and I pay them above average wages. That's quid pro quo. I pay for what I get. But what do I do when, as a group or a team, the staff performs beyong my expectations of "above average"? That requires an additional compensation, and that's what I call "sharing the profits" or a bonus. It is only given when earned, so how could I possibly give it with resentment or grudgingly?

I'm going to explain how our system works, not so that you will think yours has to be that way, but just to give you an idea of one that works.

About five years ago, I froze all salaries in the practice at a certain level for each particular job. Entry level employees could earn salary increases up to that level, but when they reached the maximum, that was it on salary increases. Every eighteen months, I look at the maximum salary for each job description to see if it's still "above average" for our area, and I make any necessary adjustments. All compensation above salary comes through bonus money, and our system works like this:

The practice is willing to pay 22 percent of its monthly collections for the combination of salaries and bonuses. Let's assume that we collect $30,000 for the month. Twenty-two percent of $30,000 is $6,600. Let's also assume that the total of all staff salaries is $5,200. Subtracting the salaries from the $6,600 leaves $1,400 to be divided as bonus money. Since bonus money is earned as a function of team effort, it is divided equally among all staff members. The entry level receptionist (after a six-month probation time) gets the same bonus check as the 18-year veteran hygienist. So in our hypothetical month, each staffer would get a $200 bonus.

Why do I say that bonus money is earned as a function of team effort? If the system is based on "collections," what does the chairside assistant have to do with that? Well, if she's not assisting the doctor so as to be maximally productive, the front desk people don't have as much to collect, and if the hygienists aren't being aware of openings in the doctor's schedule and filling them in with possiblities from their hygiene patients, and if everyone isn't generating referrals, collections will surely be affected.

The system is simple and fair and has some extra benefits to the practice. It is predictable. I know, at the beginning of the year, that staff salaries and bonuses will be 22 percent of whatever we collect, and I can count on that in my planning. I also have the assurance that the staff will not ask to bring on another employee unless (a) they really need help and (b) the new person will add to the productivity of the practice. The staff knows that if they bring on another person, that salary will be added in to the total of staff salaries and will reduce the bonus pool. So I know that they would rather all work a bit harder

rather than add to the staff, and as long as the job get
care how the 22 percent gets split up.

What happens if a staff member isn't pulling her shar
to get her bonus? That has happened, and it was handled among the
staff. They held a meeting, let that staff member know that she wasn't
contributing to the overall productivity, and that they had decided that
she would be on a one-month probation–without a bonus–and then
they would meet again. That worked like a charm. The probationer
got right back into the game, and there hasn't been a problem since.

FINDING THE RIGHT STAFF
AND KEEPING THEM

As if dentistry hasn't had enough crisis in the past ten years (not to
mention the AIDS problem), a new one is developing that will
ultimately threaten every dental practice. For a variety of reasons
(which are beyond the scope of this book), young people are not
choosing to enter the fields of dental assisting and dental hygiene.

Ten or fifteen years ago, when I ran an ad for an assistant or
receptionist or even hygienist in a local paper, I got 25 or 30 responses,
did a lot of "interviewing" on the phone, whittled the field down to four
or five, and called them in for face-to-face interviews. I recall that very
often my dilemma was in trying to choose between two or three really
good people. Back then, when I advertised for "experience only" or
"certified only," that's who called. Back then, in our area, we had three
colleges and two junior colleges teaching dental assisting, and three
dental schools teaching full classes of hygienists.

Now-a-days, an ad for any position often goes completely unan-
swered, and when we do receive responses, they are more than likely
unexperienced, let alone certified. Only two of our dental schools are
teaching hygiene, and their classes are far from filled. None of our local
colleges or junior colleges is teaching assisting any longer, due to
dramatic drops in enrollment. The State of Maryland has decreed that
only a Certified Dental Assistant may perform any of the procedures
that today's practitioner requires of an assistnat. And yet, apparently,
dentistry's historic reluctance to pay decent wages and provide
adequate benefits, coupled with the increased risk factor of exposure
to hepatitis and AIDS-related diseases, has finally come to roost and
made the dental profession of little interest to qualified entry-level
career choosers.

The problem is bound to get much worse before it gets better, and
the only real solution I can see is to raise the salaries and the images

of the people we rely on to run our practices. That will obviously take time, and the commitment to follow that approach hasn't even been adequately debated in the dental societies yet. Clearly, the practitioner "out on the front line" trying to run a practice can't wait for long-term solutions.

Until our profession comes to grips with this potentially devastating situation, the individual dentist will have to find interim solutions. If the crisis has already hit your practice, I suggest the following steps:

First, you need to make your practice "attractive" to potential employees. By that I mean it needs to develop the reputation in your community as "the" place to work. In order to run the kind of practice that is capable of surviving and thriving, you need to have quality people on your team, and the days are long since gone when we can attract quality people with minimal salaries and puny benefits. I have always paid my employees better than anyone else, and people who work in dentistry in my area know that. At times, we've had good people waiting for an opening on the staff. Our practice also offers a full package of enticing and competitive benefits. Based on our reputation, when we do have an opening and no one "in the wings," very often by just putting the word out in the dental community we will shake someone loose who is unhappy in his or her present circumstances. I hope that doesn't sound like "stealing" employees, but it's done all the time in other businesses, and under today's circumstances, the practice that is willing to adequately compensate quality employees deserves to get them.

With a dwindling number of qualified and experienced people in the dental job pool, I believe that more and more of us will have to return to the system that I used in the early days of my career. Back in the early sixties, there were very few trained assistants around. What most us did then, and what I think many of us will have to resort to in the near future, is "on the job training."

I read an article recently by a well-known business consultant, who made the statement that McDonald's was really not in the fast food business–they were really in the "people training" business. What he meant was that the real success of the McDonald empire has more to do with the well- trained people who run the stores than with the quality of the food they serve. McDonald's has a very sophisticated and very efficient training program that is capable of turning the lowest entry level job applicants into courteous and well-disciplined employees. I really believe that the good dental practices will have to get into the "people training" business in order to survive. What that will mean and how it will look in each practice will vary, of course. In a well-established practice with a good existing staff, the recruitment, selection, and training of new people should be a staff function. In a young practice, the dentist will have to assume that responsibility. In either case, assuming that fewer job applicants will have experience or skills, the criteria for selection must be personality and willingness to learn. Of our current staff of six, three were castoffs from other practices, and all three were let go for being "disruptive elements." Their real problem was boredom. They were dying to take on responsibility, and no one would give them any. Today, they literally run my practice. They're happy as clams and so am I.

Until our profession takes the necessary steps to make working in dentistry appealing to young people, successful practices will have to make themselves attractive, and then hire "people-oriented" people, and then be willing to train them on the job. Even that approach will not solve the shortage of dental hygienists. The short-term answer to that problem seems to be the hiring of recent dental graduates as hygienists/minor periodontal therapists. Staff retention is a direct reflection of a practice's ability to meet the needs of and to give recognition to valuable employees. In today's work world, people have a definite need for a voice in the decision-making process. They also need to be fairly compensated for their commitment and dedication, and they deserve to be well taken care of by their place of employment. We truly can't do the job without them, and they deserve to know that, too, and to be acknowledged for their contribution to the profession. People who work in that type of environment tend to stick around.

THE TEAM IN BAD TIMES

I think I've made the point that I take good care of the people I work with. Their salaries are at the high end of the range in our geographic area. They receive bonuses as their share in the profits of the practice, and they participate in a full variety of fringe benefits. The practice is incorporated, and we have a pension plan. The practice also pays for employee health insurance, continuing education, and uniforms.

About three years ago, in a meeting with the accountant, he let me know that employee costs had gotten out of hand. In spite of a good year as far as production and collection were concerned, my net profit increase over the previous year had been puny. We then discussed what changes would have to be made in order to bring things back into line. To make those changes, I had to ask the staff to give up some things that they had become accustomed to. I gave myself some time to think the matter through and finally decided that this was not "my" problem; it was a "practice" problem, and I needed to discuss it with my partners.

At the next staff meeting, I let them know what the accountant had told me: that, in spite of a good year, my slice of the pie had hardly increased, while they had continued to share in the profits. I let them know that if the tables were turned–that if we would have had a good year and I would have hogged the profits–they would feel the way that I do. I then went on to explain how some of the systems of compensation that we had set up years before had gotten out of hand, and that they needed to be adjusted to make the system fair to me, as well as to them. I also told them that I thought they all knew me well enough to know that I have always been generous in sharing the goodies of the practice, and that it was not easy for me to take things away, rather than to give. I then laid out the details: a change in the form of the pension plan that would give me a greater portion of the assets; a change in the bonus system that would decrease the percentage that they got to split among themselves; and a cap on the dollar amount for their health care insurance.

I then suggested that I leave the room for awhile so they could discuss this matter by themselves. It took about ten minutes for them to call me back in. The Office Manager spoke for the staff and said, "Dr. Ehudin, nobody likes to take a cut in income or in benefits, but we know that you've always been fair with us, and we know that if you feel like you're not getting your fair share out of the practice it's going to affect how you work with us, and in the long run we'll suffer from it anyway. So we just figured out that the only way around this is for us to make sure the practice just keeps doing better, so we can all keep doing better."

And that was it.

What I learned from that experience was that if you are good and fair with your employees when times are good, you can count on them to be with you if times get bad.

I know that the story I just told was not about "bad times," but the message was clear to me. Based on their reaction to that situation, I feel confident that should the economy slow down or worse, I could rely on my partners to work it out together. If hard times should really come, I can't think a more consoling thought than to know that I won't be in it alone. If profits are down and we're struggling to pay the bills, rather than my being burdened with trying to keep the staff, they will actually be in the thick of it with me, trying to work it out. The good will that has built up in the good times may well be the number one factor in getting us, as a practice, through the hard times.

Before ending this discussion of the dental team, I want to say a word about "fun." We have a lot of fun in our office. We do a lot of dentistry, and we do it well, and we have fun, too. And I think that's an important element in the concept of team. If a group of people in the work place like each other, are challenged by what they are doing, and derive a sense of accomplishment from their achievements, it's just natural that they'll have a good time together. Most of our fun takes place behind the scenes (out of range of our patients), but enough of it spills out into the treatment areas that patients get a sense that we enjoy our work and each other, and I think people are turned on by that. Yes, we take our profession seriously, and yes, there must be an appropriateness to the kind of fun we have in the office, but we find that a healthy dose of humor can actually help our patients to relax and make their treatment easier. If you're not having any fun in your practice, I doubt if anyone else is.

CHAPTER SEVEN

THE HYGIENE PROGRAM –
the Heartbeat of Your Practice.

U nquestionably, we general dentists have come to recognize that a well-run hygiene program is vital to the overall success of our practices under normal economic conditions. It also doesn't take much imagination to predict that when times get tough for our patients, a reflex response will be to put off or delay elective procedures. With fewer discretionary dollars available, patients will be looking for corners to cut, and since most of what we consider to be the "gravy" of our production falls into that category, we can expect to be doing less crown and bridge and cosmetic dentistry. Patients will be looking at all of their expenses and looking to do the bare necessity. What that bare necessity happens to be, as far as dentistry is concerned, will have a lot to do with how well you and your staff have educated and motivated your patients, particularly in the area of oral hygiene.

If you have stressed the importance of good hygiene and of regular scaling and polishing as the key to a healthy dentition, and if your patients are prevention oriented and understand and appreciate the value of routine care, that kind of care will perhaps become the "bare necessity," but they will stay with it.

Keeping your practice hygiene production healthy in good times may well be what keeps your practice going if times become hard.

As part of a "holding action" for all of your patients, maintaining the periodontal system in good health is a strategy that every educated patient will comprehend. If you are able to hold your recall system together in hard times, you have a fighting chance to keep your overall production at an acceptable level. In a well-run practice, 30 to 40 percent of the doctor's production comes from the hygiene recall system. If patients are dropping out of the recall system, it won't be long before not only hygiene production suffers, but the practice as a whole.

In good economic times, the efficiency of the recall or patient retention system can be used to measure the quality of the care you and your staff are providing. People go back to a place where they've been well taken care of. In bad times, the efficiency of the recall system can be a measure of the practice's ability to survive. If you wait until hard times are upon you, it will certainly be too late to do much about your patient retention system.

The time to fine tune your recall system is now.

But before you can make any necessary adjustments, you'll need to know how your system is functioning at present. The method I recommend for system evaluation is not perfect, but it can give you a pretty good idea of how you are doing.

You begin by taking count of your active patient charts. Assuming that most patients will have two recall visits per year, double that number to get the total number of recall appointments per year. Then look to see how many recall visits you actually had last year. Setting up a ratio will give you the percentage effectiveness of your system.

For example:
- You have 1,000 active patient charts.
- That equals 2,000 recall visits per year.
- Last year you had 1,600 recall visits in hygiene.
- That's 80 percent effectiveness.

Another place to look is at recall cards. Obviously, you should have one for every active patient. A count will reveal any discrepancy, and every missing card represents a patient who has "fallen through the cracks" and is lost from your practice.

So let's look at the mechanics of an effective recall system. First, I've found that it's vital to the success of whatever system is being used that one person be responsible for it. That doesn't mean that he or she must "do" the system, but it does mean that that person is responsible and answerable for the success of the system. In our practice, the hygienist is responsible for making the system work. When it does, she gets the credit; when it doesn't, she has to get it working again. She doesn't have to work it alone, and actually gets help from several other staffers, but she is held accountable for the system's effectiveness.

Years ago, we used a system of sending out postcards to patients, letting them know that they were due for a checkup. It was then up to the patient to give us a call and set up an appointment. I suppose that system was better than no system at all, but not much.

We got smart when we realized that "a bird in the hand" was the only one we could really count on, and an appointment "on the book" was worth much more than a promise to make one. So we make the patient's next recall appointment right away. The hygienist actually does it at the end of her recall visit with each patient.

HERE'S HOW IT WORKS:

We use a "split" hygiene appointment book. It's a ring binder so pages can be taken out and put back in. The current three months stay at the front desk and are used for confirming patients, changing the schedule when needed, and working with "present" hygiene appointments.

The next three months are kept in the back with the hygienist. So when Gail is finished with her patient and is waiting for me or has a spare minute, she asks the patient if "Wednesday at 10 a.m." is a good time for her. If she says "Yes", then Gail says, "Let's go ahead and save you that time for your next recall visit," and she makes the appointment. She fills in that time and date on a postcard, has the patient address it to herself, and files it under the previous month to be mailed out. Having the hygienist make the appointment has several advantages. Aside from giving a measure of control to the person responsible for the system, there is real "power" in having the patient make an appointment directly with the person he or she will be seeing. This system also gives the hygienist flexibility regarding how long an appointment she wants next time and at what interval–six months? four? three? The postcard that the patient filled out will be mailed three weeks prior to the appointment, and we call to confirm two days before. Ninety percent of our patients make their next appointment that way, and most of them keep the one they made.

If they get the card five months later and realize they'll be out of town that day, they can call and set a new time. This is important: If a patient cancels a recall appointment (or any appointment, for that matter) and doesn't make another one, his name, phone number, and the kind of appointment go into the "Pending Book." More about that in a moment. So every patient either has an appointment for recall or is in

Don't Let This Happen To You . . .
It's Time For Your Dental Check-up!

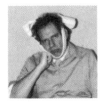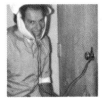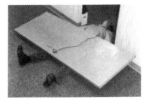

MORTON M. EHUDIN, DDS
9500 LIVINGSTON ROAD • FORT WASHINGTON, MARYLAND 20744
301 248-2020

Fig. 7–1 Reminder Postcard

the Pending Book. No one falls through the cracks. Those patients who try to fall through the cracks are sent, what we call, our "funny postcard." It's the most effective approach we've ever used to bring stray sheep back into the fold (Fig.7–1). Well, how about the patients who don't want to make a next appointment? They address a card to themselves reminding them that they are due, and it will be mailed out in the month before, and they go into the Pending Book. The rule is: either an appointment or the Pending Book. The same rule applies to patients who need work to be done. They either make an appointment, or they are entered into the Pending Book. The Pending Book becomes the receptionist's best friend when she has to fill in a cancellation or a changed appointment.

In examining the hygiene aspect of your practice, it's improtant for you to understand that 80 percent effectiveness for recall system does not mean that your hygiene department is 80 percent effective. To evaluate overall hygiene effectiveness, it's necessary to add into the equation the new patient hygiene visits. So if you saw 250 new patients last year, we can assume they accounted for 375 visits (the new patients seen in January through June would have two visits for the year, and those seen after July would have only one). That 375 added to the 1,600 recall visits equals 1,975 hygiene visits for the year. If your hygienist sees an average of 9 patients per day, 5 days a week , 48 weeks a year, she has available 2,160 visits per year. The ratio of available visits to actual visits shows the hygiene department to be operating at 91 percent effectiveness – close enough to capacity that hiring another hygienist is a realistic consideration.

Why am I bothering to do so much statistical evaluation on hygiene? Because in order to have an effective hygiene department in your practice, you need to rid yourself of some myths and use a rational approach to making decisions for the good of your practice. Questions like "When should I get a hygienist?" and "Should she be part-time or full-time, or just how much time?" have been traditionally answered "seat of the pants." I think you can see how a statistical breakdown of your patient load (both recall and new patients) can tell you, rather accurately, how many days of hygiene your practice needs.

For the busier practice, that kind of statistical analysis can tell the doctor when a second hygienist is required. Do you know when most practices take on a second hygienist? When the first one seems to be "booked up." And how many practitioners never consider a second hygienist just because their hygienists are "booked up"? If a practice statistically needs eight days a week of hygiene and only has one hygienist, of course she will be "booked up." But you can see that there is no way that that practice's recall system can be very effective. Lots of patients must be falling through the cracks. If the doctor doesn't do a statistical analysis of his practice's hygiene needs, he would never know that was happening. As far as he's concerned, "The hygienist is real busy, so everything must be fine."

Who made the rule that a dentist should only have one hygienist? Who said we couldn't have two, or three, or four, or five if our patient load justified that number? If you'll take the time to do an analysis of your true hygiene needs, I think you'll be surprised to discover what they really are, compared to what you think they are.

One of the quickest and easiest ways to increase your practice volume and productivity is to determine your real hygiene needs and then provide them.

That means statistically evaluating how many days of hygiene you need, and then providing the space and manpower to get the job done, and then setting up monitoring the recall system to give all of your patients the kind of preventive care you want them to have.

With the decline of caries as a disease factor in dentistry, the practice of the future will obviously center around prevention, especially of periodontal disease. It's not difficult to imagine the dental practice of tomorrow with a staff of five or six hygienists providing routine care to a large number of patients, and the doctor supervising that care and providing restorative care as perhaps 20 or 30 percent of the total productivity of the practice.

Similarly, in hard economic times, a practice with an effective hygiene program can go a long way toward compensating for a decrease in elective dental procedures.

A PROPHY IS NOT A PROPHY IS NOT A PROPHY

In the process of evaluating and restructuring and reorienting your hygiene department, I believe it's also important to rethink some of the basis notions that most of us have about hygiene.

Some questions to consider are:

- Who made up the law that people should have their teeth cleaned every six months?
- Who said that a "cleaning" should take 20 minutes or half an hour or 45 minutes?
- Who dictated that every "cleaning" must be accompanied by an examination?
- Who gave us the rule that a "six-month checkup" should consist of scaling and polishing?

Before I attempt to respond to the questions I've posed, some historical background:

As part of my dental education, I was taught to manipulate dental floss, but was also given the warning that it was "for professional use only." Believe it or not, in the late fifties it was common knowledge that human beings did not possess adequate manual dexterity to floss their own teeth. I was told that if people tried to use floss they would "do more harm than good." I know that sounds absurd today, but 30 years ago, it was "the truth"–until Bob Barkley came along and convinced the profession that people weren't all that fumble-fingered and could actually be taught to clean their teeth with a piece of string.

That revelation was the beginning of what we now consider to be good oral hygiene instruction. And, like most of my conscientious collagues, I began teaching and preaching the virtues of daily flossing. After nearly 20 years of hard work in this area, I've come to two conclusions: (a) Bob Barkley was right.   Just about everyone has enough manual dexterity to manipulate dental floss safely between their teeth, and (b) in all honesty, I believe that no more than 20 to 25 percent of my patients really floss their teeth on a daily basis.

Having faced up to that reality, I realized the futility and the foolishness of our six-month scoldings, urgings, and scare tactics. The truth was that some people were going to floss and some just were not–

no matter what we did or didn't do. (And take my word for it, in 20 years we tried every motivational approach that anybody suggested and some that we thought up ourselves.)

Here's the conclusion I came to about a year ago: If a patient won't (or can't) take care of his mouth adequately, we'll give him the option of letting us do it for him. So now, when one of my hygienists sees a patient who obviously isn't using proper oral hygiene technique, she'll say something like this:

> "Mr. Brown, you've been a patient of ours for over five years now, and you come in every six months for your cleanings, and every time you tell me that you haven't been doing your flossing and brushing the way I've shown you. And then I show you again and you say you're going to do it, but the truth is it's not getting done, and what suffers is the health of your gums. They're just not looking the way they're supposed to, so I want to give you a couple of choices. One is that we make another try at getting you to clean your teeth the way I know would work, and the other is just to have me do more frequent cleanings and keep your gums healthy that way."

Would it surprise you to learn that the vast majority of patients presented with those options select the more frequent cleanings with a great sense of relief? Instead of "beating up" on patients who weren't doing things "our way," we've given them an alternative that accomplishes our purpose (to achieve the best possible level of periodontal health for each patient) and frees them from the biannual guilts.

As a pleasant side effect, we've added more potential hygiene to our hygiene workload. When we do our analysis now, we know that doubling our patient numbers (two visits per year) is inaccurate. We have a growing number of patients that we see four, five, or even six times a year.

Our most recent analysis indicates that we should start looking for that third hygienist soon, and as our hygiene department grows so does the quality of the service we render. Our hygienists get to custom design a hygiene program for each patient that works best for them. Gone are the days of the "standard" appointment. Patients are appointed for an amount of time appropriate to their individual needs (and charged accordingly). We're more and more getting away from calling those visits "recall" and thinking more and more in terms of "continuing care." Unlike the "prophy" appointment, I'm only called in to do an examination biannually, and rather than being limited to scaling and polishing, our hygienists use whatever means are necessary to bring that particular patient to a state of health – be it flouride treatments, irrigations, pH testing, diet counseling, etc. All of that begins with the new patient examination. In the past, when a new patient was scheduled for a first visit in our office, it was an appointment with the hygienist for a series of x-rays, an examination, and a "cleaning." Now, new patients almost never see the hygienist on the first visit. They come for x-rays, an examination, and a consultation. It's at that first visit that we determine what kind of hygiene appointment or appointments they'll need. When new patients insist, on the phone, that they have a "cleaning" on their first visit, our receptionist asks what kind of cleaning they need. Obviously, they can't answer that question, and Dottie tells them we don't know either until the doctor has examined them.

I'm sure you've had the same problem in your practice that we had in ours, if you tried to do a "cleaning" on that first visit. If the hygienist spent 30 minutes cracking off a 10-year deposit of calculus behind the lower anteriors, and then said, "Mrs. Green, I've still got a lot to do to get your teeth clean. I'll need to get you back in again," there's a good chance that Mrs. Green was thinking either "She's slow and couldn't get finished in time" or "She's just trying to get me back so she can charge another fee." Our new approach totally eliminates that awkward situation.

At the first visit, after doing the examination, I determine if the patient will need a routine prophylaxis (for the patient with minimum deposits, good oral hygiene, and healthy tissue), a double appointment (for the patient who has gone for more than a year with no dental care and moderate deposits), or the new patient periodontal series. If I think a patient will need the series, I call in one of the hygienists to meet the patient, have a look at the situation, and explain the series (Fig. 7–2).

The periodontal series was designed for the type of new patient that we formerly referred out to the periodontist immediately after doing the examination, until I found out that the first thing the periodontist did was to turn the patient over to his hygienist for a series of scalings. Now, I'll match either of my hygienists against any of the ones working in our local periodontist's offices, so I didn't see why we couldn't do that first phase of treatment "at home" in our office.

When we identify a new patient that needs the series, here's what the hygienist tells him:

COWARDS

Dr. Morton M. Ehudin
Livingston Square Mall
9500 Livingston Road
Fort Washington, Maryland 20744
248-2020

Gum Disease Control Program

Gum disease (periodontal disease) does not happen overnight.
It is a slow deterioration of the gum around the tooth which, if left untreated, will eventually affect the tooth's bony support. As the bond around a tooth weakens, the tooth becomes loose and sore, and will ultimately be lost.

The signs of gum disease are:

1. Bleeding gums   4. Bad breath
2. Red, puffy gums   5. Loose teeth
3. Sore, tender gums   6. Pus around teeth

The purpose of our Gum Disease Control Program is to "put out the fire" of gum disease. Over the five appointments in the program, we will be working with you to eliminate the symptoms of bleeding, redness and tenderness. When you no longer have bleeding, and your gums are pink and healthy-looking, we will reevaluate. If the problem involved only the gums, we'll set up your next cleaning appointment for three months later, and then eventually work back into a six month schedule. If, however, the evaluation shows deep pockets around the teeth or loss of bone, we'll be making recommendations to handle those problems.

It is important for you to know that gum disease cannot be cured by the dentist or the hygienist alone. It is really a joint effort. All the "cleanings" in the world are worthless unless you do your part. Gum disease can be stopped and controlled, but it takes work. You have to become an oral hygiene fanatic. (You know-the kind of person who *even* flosses after lunch!)

So, if you're willing to work with us, together we can make your mouth healthy again, and give you every assurance of keeping your teeth.

Fig. 7–2 Explanation of Periodontal Series

"Mr. White, from the examination that Dr. Ehudin did, it's clear to us that you've got a pretty bad gum problem. There's a good chance that you'll eventually have to see a gum specialist to have your problem cured, but we want to see if we can get most, if not all, of your gum disease under control right here, and the way we'll do that is to set up a series of five appointments with me. At the first one, I'll be doing some measurements and recordings so we can evaluate our progress as we go along, and then I'll start removing the hard food deposits around your teeth. The next three visits will be for very carefully getting all of those hard deposits off and trying to get your gums to heal up back against the teeth. By the fifth visit, all the bleeding you have now should be gone, and your gums should have no more swelling and should be nice and pink, instead of that angry red color. So at that last visit in the series, I'll remeasure everything and polish your teeth, and then together with Dr. Ehudin, we'll decide if you need any more treatment, or if we can start our continuing care."

SUMMARY

In light of the changes occurring in dentistry in general, and specifically in light of the possibility of difficult economic times ahead, practices that have fully developed their hygiene and prevention programs will have the best chance to survive and actually thrive in the years to come.

ACTIVE STEPS TO
UPGRADE YOUR HYGIENE DEPARTMENT

1. Stop doing "cleanings" on new patients' first appointments.
2. Start viewing hygiene as double phased – treatment and continuing care – and charge appropriately.
3. Custom tailor treatment and maintenance to suit the individual patient.
4. Stop "beating up" on patients who won't stick to your oral hygiene criteria.
5. Monitor the statistics of your hygiene program and design a program to fit your practice's needs.
6. Institute a recall system that is trackable and effective.

CHAPTER EIGHT

SPECIALITIES – NO LONGER SO SPECIAL

T he development of the specialties during my professional lifetime has taken some interesting turns, and I believe that if difficult economic times do come, they will resume their proper role in dentistry.

Was there life before the specialties? What was the practice of dentistry like before there were endodontists and periodontists and pedodontists? General dentists did everything, to the best of their ability. As each of the specialty areas developed advanced skills and training, the general dentist became aware that there were colleagues available to him and his patients for procedures that were beyond his own training and capability. It was probably no coincidence that the rapid growth of the specialties corresponded with the "Golden Age of Dentistry." In the 1950s and 1960s, the ratio of practitioners to population was so favorable that every dentist had more than enough patients to see and dentistry to do. In that "sellers market" the general practitioner was only too happy to refer to a specialist not just the difficult case or the difficult patient, but very often, for convenience sake, all of the "specialty" treatment that came his way. With an overabundance of patients, most G.P.'s were content to make a living doing the operative dentistry and the prosthetics and leave the endo and ortho and perio and surgery to the specialists.

That arrangement seemed to work well for all concerned in the Golden Age, but as the schools began pumping out more dentists (and more and more specialists) just as the effects of 20 or 30 years of prevention was driving down the rate of dental disease, the cavalier attitude of "sending everything to the specialist" began to appear foolhardy. In today's environment, it seems crazy. In the future, it may well be suicidal.

In hope of not being misunderstood, let me say that I am not anti-specialist. I'm happy to have them around–for their intended purpose. I believe specialists should be doing "special" treatment. They should be doing difficult or unusual procedures or treating difficult or unusual patients. They should not be involved in the routine aspects of treatment. I am also not advocating that untrained generalists begin extracting impacted third molars, treating severe malocclusions, and doing bone grafts.

What I do strongly believe is that within each of the specialty areas there are procedures that (with proper training) should be undertaken by the general dentist. And perhaps "should" is too weak a term for the unstable future. If times get bad, the general dentist "must" be able to treat a wide range of problems heretofore left to the specialists.

Any generalist will verify that patients have a strong resistance to being "referred out." How often when making a referral have we heard, "But, Doctor, can't you do it here?" That reluctance is based on the trust established with the doctor and the anxiety of being sent somewhere where they may not be as well taken care of. In a down economy, that hesitance may be compounded by financial consider-ations. Patients with money problems may be looking to the general dentist to treat them at a more reasonable cost.

From the G.P.'s point of view, it may well become economically unfeasible to send treatment out of the office that could stay "at home." In the face of decreased revenues from "elective" procedures in the prosthetic and cosmetic areas, the generalist must take a hard look at what and how much dentistry he is referring out. The time to take that look and do something about it is not when hard times come. The time is now!

If you agree with my assessment, you can't wait until we are deep in a recession to take a course on upgrading your surgical skills or learning to do molar endodontics. You need to do that right now and have a couple of years of experience under your belt when those skills could come to mean the difference between financially making it or not in your practice.

Now I'm going to climb somewhat out on a limb and spell out specifically what I believe a general dentist should be capable of competently handling in his practice, in each of the specialty areas. Please notice, I said "competently." If you lack competence in any of the following areas, there are excellent continuing education courses all over the country to bring you up to that level. I've listened to specialists tell stories, with obvious glee, of botched treatment by incompetent G.P.'s. Some of those may well be true, but I've seen a lot of "specialty" treatment done by generalists that was outstanding, and I can't help but believe that some of those "horror stories" are clumsy attempts to keep the G.P.'s nose buried in amalgam.

ORAL SURGERY

I believe it should be within the competence of every G.P. to incise and drain an abscess. I believe that every generalist should be capable of doing routine extractions, including flapping and the removal of fractured roots and root tips, and the surgical preparation of ridges for dentures. I think G.P.'s should be able to remove erupted and partially erupted third molars and most soft tissue impactions of same. I believe that generalists should have the ability to perform a biopsy of oral tissues.

I think the oral surgeons should be dealing with the predetermined difficult extraction cases, the medically compromised patients, orthognathic surgery, and trauma cases. That's what they've been trained to do, and that should be their function within the profession.

ENDODONTICS

Certainly, the general dentist should be doing 90 percent of the endodontic cases in his practice. He should be able to handle all but the most difficult or unusual anterior teeth, as well as the bicuspids, and at least 75 percent of the molars. In recent years, techniques and materials in the field of endodontics have made major strides toward bringing competent and efficient root canal therapy within the scope of every G.P. The principles of good endodontics are the same, be they for a central incisor or an upper second molar, and there are many fine courses teaching endo for the general dentist. It is certainly time to put old prejudices aside and at least make a reevaluation after looking into today's world of endodontics.

PERIODONTICS

I believe that not only for financial reasons, but also from a professional point of view, the general dentist is obliged to take his patient through the first phase of periodontal therapy. Gone are (and should be) the days when the patient with periodontal problems presented to the generalist and was, immediately after examination, "shipped off to the periodontist" – often never to be seen again. Gone are (and should be) the days when the periodontist took over not only the periodontal therapy, but the overall treatment planning for the referred patient.

The general dentist, with proper training, should develop a comprehensive plan of treatment and carry the patient through the initial stages of his periodontal planning. That should, I believe, include an in-depth explanation of the causes and consequences of periodontal disease, thorough oral hygiene instructions, and removal of all supra- and sub-gingival deposits through scaling, root planing, and curettage. Using those skills, the generalist should be capable of bringing the disease under control (i.e., no bleeding on probing and tissue non-edematous and healthy in appearance). Since it is impossible to reach that state of periodontal health without the full cooperation of the patient, only patients who have participated in controlling their own disease process should be referred for more complex periodontal procedures. To do otherwise is a waste of the patient's time and money and of the periodontist's skills. The incorporation of advanced periodontal procedures into an overall plan of treatment, at the request of the generalist and for a patient who has demonstrated responsibility for her own health, puts the periodontist into the support role that the designation "specialist" infers.

ORTHODONTICS

Obviously, skeletal malocclusions, gross tooth size to arch size discrepancies, and complex orthodontic procedures should be treated by orthodontists. But there remains a wide range of orthodontic procedures that are well within the capabilities of the general dentist. Closing diastimas in normal occlusions, correcting anterior cross bites, and correcting "flared" anterior teeth prior to the restoration of lost posterior vertical dimension are manageable by the generalist.

Certainly, in this age of prevention, the G.P. has a role to play in interceptive orthodontics. For five years now, I've had excellent success using Dr. Earl Bergerson's Occlus-o-guide system in diagnosing and resolving developing orthodontic problems in my young patients. His course is excellent, and his technique should be in the armamentarium of every general dentist who sees children. Especially in hard economic times, the general practitioner should have available to him a less costly and effective alternative to waiting for the "full blown" orthodontic problem to develop, and then having no option but "braces." For many families, it may well come down to "whatever the G.P. can do" or nothing.

PEDIATRIC DENTISTRY

I've never understood the general dentist who doesn't see children. Aside from the pleasures of interacting with young people, taking care of children is the backbone of a family practice. If you have eliminated children from your practice, and we fall upon hard times, many families on reduced incomes may take a hard look at the "luxury" of sending their kids to a pedodontist and turn to you to treat their whole family. I know that many G.P.'s regard seeing children as "unproductive" or "too stressful" or even "disruptive," and I don't mind if you come to think of it as a "loss leader," but I urge you to reexamine your pediatric referrals in light of the general philosophy I've put forth here. If you're referring out the three and four years olds with large carious lesions and the difficult management cases, fine. But if you are routinely referring out children, I suggest you reconsider and develop whatever skills you are lacking to bring and hold "all" of the family in your practice. If your adult patients, for financial reasons, ask you to take care of the children and you can't or won't, they may well go elsewhere–as a family.

Do I seem to be asking too much of the general dentist? Is it too much to expect him to expand his abilities in all of the "specialty" areas? Let me clearly state that I'm not suggesting moving on all fronts simultaneously. But surely, over a period of one to three years, using a well-thought-out plan of good continuing education, any G.P. can learn the procedures and techniques I've discussed. Aside from the satisfaction derived from expanding your horizons, the financial health of your practice may come to rest on your ability to treat more "in house" if times get tough.

CONTINUING EDUCATION

Over the years, I've developed some very strong feelings about continuing education. As a young dentist, I used to believe that I was continuing my dental education by attending sessions of my local society. I don't mean to knock their programs, and I'm certain that I learned a lot by attending those meetings, but I was totally passive in receiving that kind of learning. Whatever was on the program was what I got. I still go to the meetings, but it's more of a "fill in."

Now I look at continuing education by asking myself the question,

"What do I need to learn next, either for myself or for the good of the practice?" And then, when I've answered, I go out and find the best course or source in the country that provides what I need. And I'm willing to go anywhere and pay any price. That's what I call "real" continuing education.

One final note: If I were a young dentist, just beginning my career, there would be two organizations that I would use to guide my professional life. For technical advancement and a philosophy of dentistry and of life, I would take every course at the Pankey Institute in Coral Gables, Florida. For practice management and financial planning, I would associate myself with Dr. Michael Schuster's Center for Professional Development in Scottsdale, Arizona. With that combination on your side, success in dentistry is about as sure as anything in life can be.

CHAPTER NINE

ADVANCED PLANNING

As a part of this chapter on advanced planning, I've deemed it prudent to take a look at a "worst case" scenario, not to create apprehension, but to stimulate thought and to assist you in planning for the future.

How will hard economic times affect your practice? Any answer to that question can only be speculative, but some possibilities seem more certain than others, and in trying to prepare ourselves for what may lie ahead, making some educated guesses can lead us in the right direction.

Obviously, the scenario will vary from area to area in the country, and hard times will have more severe repercussions in some regions of the country than others. It seems safe to say that the general condition would not change overnight, although overnight changes could happen. Major government actions, for example, could be taken with no advance notice. If the banks are closed, we will all wake up one morning to find that we have no access to our accounts, or that there is a limit to withdrawals. But, generally speaking, I would imagine that the hard times would begin as a recession that would deepen, and rather than lead to a recovery, would slide into a longstanding depression. The astute professional will need to be flexible, read and interpret what's happening, and be positioned to make necessary changes.

Giving some thought to the manifestations of a depression on a general dental practice, one could anticipate some common themes:

- Unemployment will rise, and jobs and money will be harder to come by.
- Many workers will be out of work or take lower paying jobs.
- Employers will lower wages and reduce benefits.
- Dental insurance could be a sacrificed benefit.
- Patients will be increasingly reluctant or unable to use credit cards to pay for treatment.
- Patients who normally would use savings for major dental work may be reluctant to do so or may have their savings "frozen."
- Some families may lose one or both incomes.
- Job insecurity will make patients reluctant to take time off from work to keep appointments. Evening and Saturday appointments may become more in demand.
- Recall patients may stretch out the intervals between checkups.
- Parents may sacrifice their own care so the children can be taken care of.
- Patients who formerly shunned their capitation or PPO benefits and were willing to pay for "better care" may be forced to use those plans for part or all of their care.
- More patients may take the attitude, "If the insurance company doesn't pay for it, I don't want it."
- Patients will tend to put off elective procedures or want a compromise or "holding" solution.
- There will be an increased reluctance to go to a "specialist."
- Esthetics will take a back seat to function.
- Patients will want things repaired or "patched" rather than replaced.
- Long-term neglect will lead to more emergencies.
- Prevention and emergency care may become the economic backbone of the general practice.
- Competition among dentists may result in fee slashing.
- As the prices of everything go down, so will dental fees.

- Increased competition for patients may make practicing in groups more difficult, and associateships will become rare.
- Patient loyalty may erode.
- Some patients will request credit and not be able to have work done without it.
- Accounts Receivable will go up.
- Large practices may find themselves with too much space and over-staffed.
- Staff reduction or wage or benefit reductions may be necessary to bring down overhead.
- The "niceties" of practicing may have to be eliminated to keep overhead under control (flowers, coffee, newsletters, giveaways, etc.)
- Rural areas may see the return of the barter system.
- Some dental supplies may become difficult to get, and some may become unavailable.

In trying to anticipate the possible effects of hard times on our dental practices, I've attempted to cover all the scenarios from a mild short-term recession to a deep and long-standing depression. I believe that most of my recommendations, if followed through, will put your practice in the best possible position to survive and thrive in whatever economic climate we may have to face. The degree to which you may need to implement any of the steps I've suggested will of course be dictated by the severity of the economic collapse.

As I've stressed repeatedly, timely preparation is essential, and the time to begin is now–way before it appears that preparation may even be necessary. Putting your practice on a firm financial foundation, building up your volume, expanding your hygiene program, increasing your "specialty" skills, and developing the right staff all take time, and the time to begin moving along those directions is right now.

There is, however, one area of advanced planning that I will approach cautiously, both in my own practice and in making recommendations for yours. It seems reasonable to assume that in a severe economic collapse many of the supplies that we deem essential to doing business may become scarce or even unavailable. Supply items with a short shelf life leave us little option for stockpiling, but there are supplies that we must have in order to stay in operation that, at some point, may be worth accumulating. Amalgam comes to mind, and precious metals, and a certain amount of anesthetic, and gloves and masks. I'm not suggesting "hoarding," but I think some prudent "squirreling away" of supplies that will not go bad and could ultimately make the difference of your practice remaining functional is not a bad idea. How much and what supplies, I leave up to the individual practitioner.

As for overall planning, I recommend using a two-year time frame. If you approach your preparations so as to actually be "ready" two years from now, I think you can accomplish what needs to be done, and according to most economic forecasts, if hard times are ahead, they will make themselves felt about two years after a major stock market crash.

CHAPTER TEN

SUMMING UP

T his book has been written based upon some assumptions that I believe are worth taking into consideration when planning for the long range health and well-being of our dental practices. One assumption is that the "good times," as we have known them for over 50 years now, may not go on forever. There are sufficient economic signs and signals to cause the judicious practitioner to pause, evaluate the possibilities, and then take the necessary steps to insulate his practice from the changes that possibly lie ahead.

The second major assumption is that there is still adequate time to take those steps. As a dental student in the physiology laboratory, I recall an experiment that we did on a frog in a pot of tepid water. We raised the temperature of the water 1 degree every 15 minutes. The change was so slow and so subtle that the poor frog boiled before he ever realized what had happened to him. That's the way it is with slow change for humans, too. If things change ever so gradually, big changes can happen without our becoming aware. People who were carefully watching the stock market in the fall of '87 noticed some subtle shifts in the right indicators and got out before the crash. Most investors weren't watching carefully enough and got caught. Timing is everything!

The changes that we are observing now in our economy and in the international economy are strong enough signs for astute observers to predict that major change may be on the way. The careful observer will not be fooled or lulled into a false sense of security by an upswing in the market or a short-term improvement in the trade deficit or a temporary stabilization of the dollar. Looking at the big picture, any real solution to our chronic economic excesses may call upon the people of this country to "pay up" for the misuse of our credit over a long period of time. And paying up will not be pleasant. This country is too big and too strong to be destroyed by the "pay back," but we may have to go through a period of reduced expectations (at least).

Dentists who understand that must anticipate the effects of a slow, sluggish, recessionary, or even depressed economy on their practices and take appropriate steps to assure their health and possibly survival.

A practice that has its financial house in order is in far better shape to cope with a bad economy than one suffering from high receivables, poor credit policy, and out of control overhead.

A practice with a wide base of patients and a strong recall system has a better chance of survival than one with a limited number of patients and a weak system of recall.

A dentist who is capable of offering his patients a wide range of services and who is willing to offer emergency care and provide "holding action" treatment is in better position than one who does not see emergencies, is rigid in his approach to treatment, and is limited in his capabilities.

And a practitioner who tries to "go it alone" as the superstar with some "girls" will have a more difficult time than the dentist who has taken the time and effort to create a team within which he can find support and partnership.

AND FINALLY:

May the precautions of this book turn out to be unnecessary. With luck or good fortune, our economy may continue to go up and up and up, defying all laws of nature and economics. In which case, if you've followed the advice put down here, you'll only have a better, more organized, healthier, and more enjoyable practice (with a closet full of amalgam).

For whatever the future may bring, I wish you the best of everything.